7500

99BB

Fetal Autonomy
and Adaptation

Fetal Autonomy and Adaptation

Edited by

G. S. Dawes
John Radcliffe Hospital, Oxford

F. Borruto
Obstetrics and Gynaecology Clinic,
University of Verona

A. Zacutti and A. Zacutti, Jr
S. Andrea Hospital, La Spezia

JOHN WILEY & SONS
Chichester · New York · Brisbane · Toronto · Singapore

Copyright ©1990 by John Wiley & Sons Ltd.
Baffins Lane, Chichester
West Sussex PO19 1UD, England

Other Wiley Editorial Offices

John Wiley & Sons, Inc., 605 Third Avenue,
New York, NY 10158-0012, USA

Jacaranda Wiley Ltd, G.P.O. Box 859, Brisbane,
Queensland 4001, Australia

John Wiley & Sons (Canada) Ltd, 22 Worcester Road,
Rexdale, Ontario M9W 1L1, Canada

John Wiley & Sons (SEA) Pte Ltd, 37 Jalan Pemimpin 05-04,
Block B, Union Industrial Building, Singapore 2057

Library of Congress Cataloging-in-Publication Data

Fetal autonomy and adaptation/edited by G. S. Dawes,
    A. Zacutti, F. Borruto and A. Zacutti, Jr.
        p.   cm.
    Proceedings of an international workshop held Oct. 6–7, 1989,
La Spezia, Italy.
    Includes bibliographical references and index.
    ISBN 0 471 92778 3
    1. Fetus—Physiology—Congresses.
    I. Dawes, Geoffrey S.   II. Zacutti, A.
    III. Borruto, F.   IV. Zacutti A. Jr
RG610.F47   1990
612.6'47—dc20   90-12458
                                                 CIP

British Library Cataloguing in Publication Data

Fetal autonomy and adaptation.
    1. Man. Foetuses. Development
    I. Dawes, G. S.   II. Zacutti, A.
    III. Borruto, F.   IV. Zacutti, A. Jr
    612.647

    ISBN 0 471 92778 3

Phototypeset by Dobbie Typesetting Service, Tavistock, Devon
Printed and bound by Courier International, Tiptree, Colchester

Contents

Contributors

D. ARDUINI   *Clinica Ostetrica e Ginecologica, Universita Cattolica del Sacro Cuore, Policlinico A. Gemelli, Largo a Gemelli 8, 00168 Rome, Italy*

D. J. P. BARKER   *MRC Environmental Epidemiology Unit, Southampton General Hospital, Southampton, SO9 4XY, UK*

I. CETIN   *Clinica Ostetrica e Ginecologica, Ospedale San Paolo, Via A. di Rudini 8, 20142 Milan, Italy*

J. R. G. CHALLIS   *The Lawson Research Institute, St Joseph's Health Center, 268 Grosvenor Street, London, Ontario N6A 4Y2, Canada*

G. S. DAWES   *Nuffield Department of Obstetrics and Gynaecology, John Radcliffe Hospital, Oxford OX3 9DU, UK*

F. ELLENDORFF   *Institut fur Kleintierzücht, Dörnbergstrasse 25/27, Postfach 280, 3100 Celle, West Germany*

M. HANSON   *Department of Biochemistry and Physiology, University of Reading, Whiteknights, Reading, Berkshire, UK*

G. MANDRUZZATO   *Divisione di Ostetrica e Ginecologia, Istituto per L'Infanzia, Ospedale BurloGarofalo, Via dell'Istria 65, 34137 Trieste, Italy*

G. PARDI   *Clinica Ostetrica e Ginecologica, Ospedale San Paolo, Via A. di Rudini 8, 20142 Milan, Italy*

J. PATRICK (deceased)   *Department of Obstetrics, St Joseph's Hospital, 268 Grosvenor Street, London, Ontario, N6A 4Y2, Canada*

C. W. G. REDMAN   *Nuffield Department of Obstetrics and Gynaecology, John Radcliffe Hospital, Oxford OX3 9DU, UK*

G. RIZZO *Clinica Ostetrica e Ginecologica, Universita Cattolica del Sacro Cuore, Policlinico A. Gemelli, Largo a Gemelli 8, 00168 Rome, Italy*

E. SIMPSON *Cecil H. and Ida Green Center for Reproductive Biology, University of Texas, Health Science Center, S.W. Medical School, Dallas, Texas, USA*

K. THORNBURG *Department of Physiology, Oregon Health Sciences University, 3181 S.W. Sam Jackson Park Road, Portland, Oregon 97201, USA*

G. H. VISSER *Department of Obstetrics and Gynaecology, State University, 59 Oostersingel, 9713 EZ Groningen, The Netherlands*

C. WILLIAMS *Department of Paediatrics, School of Medicine, 85 Park Road, Auckland, New Zealand*

A. ZACUTTI *Ospedale Sant'Andrea, USL N19 Spezzino, Regione Liguria, Italy 19100*

Dr John Patrick, of London, Ontario, Canada
and Professor Corrado Confaloniere, secretary of the
Italian Association of Obstetricians and Gynaecologists,

who took part in the meeting in Lerici, have died. Both made
great contributions in their lifetimes and we mourn their passing.
Shelley, who loved this Italian shore, wrote:

He is made one with Nature: there is heard
His voice in all her music, from the moan
of thunder, to the song of night's sweet bird.
Adonais

Acknowledgements

We thank:

Associazione Ostetrici e Ginecologi Ospedalieri Italiani and the following industries and pharmaceutical firms for their contribution to the organization of the Workshop:

Angelini
ESAOTE Biomedica
Glaxo
Life Pharma
Pasteur Diagnostici
Shering
Tecnologie Ospedaliere
Wyeth

A particular thank-you to the Cassa di Risparmio della Spezia for their splendid Conference Center 'Villa Marigola' in San Terenzo di Lerici.

Welcome

PROFESSOR ALBERTO ZACUTTI

I would like to welcome you on behalf of the Organizing Committee, and to thank our sponsors, including the Italian Association of Hospital Obstetrics and Gynaecology.

It doesn't very often happen that so many distinguished scientists, experts in the field of fetal physiopathology and coming from all over the world, attend the same meeting. Last year Professor Dawes and I recalled the now obsolete volume *Foetal Autonomy** and so originated the idea of organizing a similar meeting, to update and discuss the problems of fetal physiopathology which have, in the meantime, been modified and improved by technical and scientific advances. That's the reason why we are here.

Present ideas on the intrauterine environment are undergoing a process of revision and discussion. We've been used to regarding the intrauterine environment as a quiet, soft and silent place, protected and free of stress. This static condition, which was considered ideal for the fetus, its autonomy and homeostasis, is well represented in Leonardo's famous picture, which reflects very accurately the anatomical character of the fetus, pictured in a quiet curled-up posture.

New ideas are spreading, according to which the intrauterine environment does not resemble this picture. On the contrary, there are several dynamic conditions to which the fetus might react with stress responses, to acoustic stimuli or light, to biochemical conditions, or to the continuous changing of the mother's emotional state as a result of the transplacental passage of chemical mediators. Another picture, reproduced from the *Comare* by Scipione Mercurio, dating back to the 16th century, is far more fantastic. It shows the fetus in an attitude of lively, frightened reaction to the stimuli reaching it (Figure 1). According to this idea, which is common, the uterus may not always be the ideal

*Wolstenholme GEW and O'Connor M (eds) (1969) *Foetal Autonomy: Ciba Foundation Symposium*. Churchill, London.

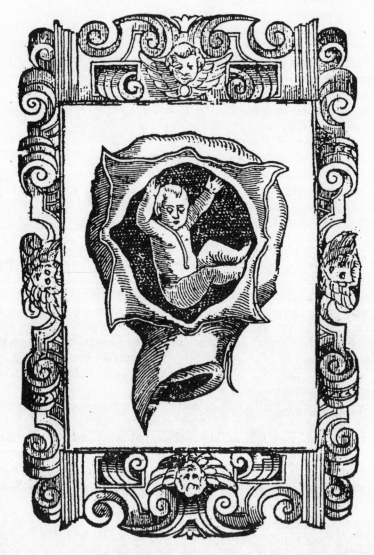

FIGURE 1   The fetus as depicted by the sixteenth century artist Scipione Mercurio in his work the *Comare*

environment for fetal life, and birth may be a rescue operation. A neonatal intensive care unit may sometimes be safer than intrauterine fetal constraint before birth.

This negative interpretation of prenatal life conditions is not new, and in my opinion arises from a cultural misunderstanding; in effect, fetal conditions are assessed in comparison with those of the adult. According to this viewpoint, the characteristics of fetal life (such as low oxygen pressure, lack of barometric pressure, presence of amniotic fluid and its inhalation, presence of environmental stimulations, and so on), instead of being considered ideal are regarded as harmful. Yet without them the fetus would stop growing or even living. The fetus has been compared with an astronaut in a spacecraft in zero gravity, or with a deep-sea diver, the umbilical cord resembling the hose which carries oxygen from the scuba to the man underwater. The diver must hold his breath with plunging, and modify his circulation and metabolism in order to withstand this unnatural condition. Speaking of 'Mount Everest in utero', as has been done several times, makes one think of the fetus as a climber breathless because of the low oxygen pressure due to altitude, without taking into consideration the fact that the fetus acquires oxygen from its mother's blood *because* of the low partial pressure of this gas in its own blood. It carries it adequately because it has a haemoglobin different from the adult, and distributes it to its own tissues through a circulation that also is quite different to the adult. For the fetus, still entirely dependent on its mother, perhaps some episodes of hypoxia may be an integral part of prenatal life. Indeed the mechanisms, which enable it to overcome such episodes easily and with no damage, are part of its normal physiology.

Even if the examples mentioned are somewhat provocative, they certainly don't give a picture of fetal life as either safe or calm enough for the baby to learn to distinguish between safety and fear; or suitable for the fetus to develop its organs mature and functionally tested in the uterus, ready to perform effectively the complex sequence of adaptations that occurs after delivery.

The reasons for the conflict between these interpretations of fetal life are several and deep. They depend essentially on the lack of a thorough knowledge of fetal physiopathology, or on the more or less conscious refusal to apply this knowledge to clinical practice. This cultural substratum, which unfortunately is widespread and deep-rooted, can lead to major consequences. Even recently, the use of sophisticated and complex fetal monitoring techniques was adopted before there was adequate knowledge of the significance to be assigned to the data which they supply. The purposes which first characterized fetal monitoring are being progressively changed. It seems that the diagnosis of hypoxia is no longer our aim; under the banner of an earlier and earlier search for signs of fetal distress, we run the risk of broadening the field too much. We pretend to a diagnostic strategy in areas so wide that they lie quite outside the problem of hypoxia. It is perhaps in this grey area, between the white of normality and the black of pathology, that we may identify that fetal function which we define as 'adaptation'. However, we do not know whether this relates to fetal conditions worsening gradually or to occasional transitory phenomena, not necessarily indicative of distress.

Professor Dawes, who conceived and organized this meeting, will act as our moderator, and in his introduction he will define the scientific purposes of our meeting.

1

Fetal Autonomy
and Adaptation

G. S. DAWES

Nuffield Department of Obstetrics and Gynaecology,
John Radcliffe Hospital, Oxford, UK

The CIBA Foundation held a meeting on Fetal Autonomy in December 1968, through the good offices of its then Director, Sir Gordon Wolstenholme, with whom I can well remember discussing the title. That meeting marked a transition point: evidence had been accumulating that the fetus, far from being a feeble diminutive version of the adult, was well able to regulate its own sophisticated affairs, many of them peculiar to itself. Indeed during the preceding two years Mont Liggins had shown that the fetus played a crucial role in the initiation of parturition in sheep. Professor Zacutti suggested that it might be appropriate to hold a meeting this year, on the 21st anniversary as near as convenient, to discuss further recent advances in fetal research. That is why we are here today.

In 1968 exploitation of the new methods for experimental observation on unanaesthetized fetuses in utero was only just beginning. Within the next few years rapid advances were made and it was recognized that, in species born precocially like the sheep and the guinea pig, there were many factors which modulated fetal behaviour from time to time. These included episodic changes in fetal state corresponding to sleep cycles postnatally, diurnal rhythms in fetal heart rate and in fetal breathing movements, changes related to maternal food intake and to the intermittent presence of uterine activity well before the onset of labour, and seasonal changes like the huge variations in plasma prolactin recently reported by Bassett et al (1988). In addition there are changes in every aspect of physiology with gestational age. There was therefore a period of reconsideration and research to measure these phenomena, and to unravel the fetal mechanisms. The use of unanaesthetized fetal animals for research has problems, in that such periodic changes must always be taken into account.

Fetal Autonomy and Adaptation. Edited by G. S. Dawes, A. Zacutti, F. Borruto and A. Zacutti, Jr
©1990 John Wiley & Sons Ltd

Observations on the human infant in utero were much facilitated by the introduction of real-time ultrasound scanning in 1975, and by the subsequent developments in ultrasound technology which allow us not only to see and measure the dimensions of the fetus and its organs, but to measure flow velocity in the blood vessels and the changing shape of the heart in systole and diastole, and to provide the visualization necessary to introduce a needle into a fetal blood vessel without excessive risk. Yet there are gaps in our ability to address questions of the human fetus in utero. Direct measurements of the blood gases are intermittent. Few measurements of intravascular pressures have been recorded, and characterization of both function and behaviour is still regrettably dependent on indirect observations. We still need the conjoint efforts of obstetricians and basic scientists in trying to unravel the mechanisms which underlie fetal autonomy. We need more and better measurements.

The title of this symposium has been chosen as Fetal Autonomy and Adaptation. Let me illustrate the subject with some examples. In general, we try to explain changes in fetal physiological function by reference to what is established knowledge in adults. But the explanations are by no means satisfactory and there is reason to believe that they may involve mechanisms of which we are as yet uncertain. We have known for many years that when an unanaesthetized fetal lamb near term is subject to isocapnic hypoxia the heart rate falls, transiently. Within 10–15 minutes it usually is close to the initial value even though the hypoxia continues. If the hypoxia is continued for an hour, not only the heart rate but also the blood pressure return to normal, though breathing movements, and movements of the fetal body and limbs, may still be much reduced. Recently several groups in Australia, Canada and the USA, have shown that if the hypoxia continues for 24 hours both breathing and fetal movements return to their normal frequency and amplitude (Bocking and Harding, 1986; Bocking et al., 1988a,b; Koos et al., 1988; Kitanaka et al., 1989). Plasma erythropoietin has risen but it is too early to expect a rise in haemoglobin concentration. There is a redistribution of cardiac output so that blood flow to the heart and brain are increased at the onset of hypoxia, and this increase persists. But if oxygen supply to the systemic arterial chemoreceptors and the brain is not returned to its initial value, then how does it come about that the behaviour of the fetus after 24 hours of hypoxia appears superficially unchanged from what it was initially? What hormonal changes take place? Can they be invoked to explain the resultant adaptation? Even in adult animals the rise in plasma erythropoietin does not persist during continued hypoxia. It would be useful if hormonal, or other such variables, could be measured as an index of persistent hypoxaemia. The obstetrician requires an unambiguous method of discriminating between hypoxaemia of short and long duration, and determining whether it is compensated or otherwise. We need to know the limits of fetal adaptation.

Changes also take place in the fetal environment. The volume of the amniotic fluid can swell or shrink, and this seems to be mainly under fetal control.

Fetal urine flow and pulmonary fluid production can be changed by fetal hormones (e.g. atrial natriuretic polypeptide and catecholamines). So we may ask whether the fetus with growth retardation and a falling amniotic fluid volume is a victim of its own adaptation. We also require some explanation of the changing function of the placenta, which not only seems to preserve its O_2 supply but also its amino-acid uptake (from the uterine or umbilical arteries) at the expense of the fetus. Is the fetus forced to adapt to preserve placental function?

Ultimately the fetus can escape, by initiating parturition. We know that, in the sheep, this is largely under fetal control. It may be a policy of last resort; do we have direct evidence that it does so happen, i.e. as a programmed response to insult? Is the timing of normal labour determined, in part or whole, by what is now recognized as the progressive fall in O_2 partial pressure in fetal arterial blood, or in O_2 supply to the placenta? Is this the explanation of some instances of premature labour in man, for instance in multiple pregnancy, if not with infection?

There are more sophisticated problems to be considered. We have difficulty in measuring the ability of the fetus, even near term, to perceive some forms of sensory stimulation. I hope someone will tell us the difference between adaptation and habituation. At first, in early gestation, we can be sure that the response to tactile stimulation is localized to the spinal cord and lower brainstem. Later, more sophisticated mechanisms come into play. But what of the response to other sensory modalities—to sound or pain, for instance? Each presents different problems in analysis and interpretation.

We also need to recall the importance of critical periods in fetal development. I will not rehearse all the many examples, from the determination of sexual behaviour in adolescence (by exposure to sex hormones *over a limited time* before or after birth according to species), to the fact that postnatal development of the visual cortex is dependent on the environment (e.g. Wiesel, 1982). Similarly removal of a whisker from the muzzle of a mouse prevents the development of the appropriate 'barrel' of neurones in the sensory cortex (Van der Loos, 1977). On the other hand there is plasticity in the rearrangement of the auditory and visual maps of the newborn ferret's world. The ferret is born in an altricial state; if an ear is plugged at birth it develops an essentially normal auditory map in the superior colliculus, in approximate register with the visual map, necessary to the accurate spatial localization of sounds (King et al., 1988; Moore et al., 1989). Development of the auditory map is affected by visual activity and information on eye position; however, there is limited capacity for the auditory map to be reorganized so that it remains aligned. We also have to remember species differences: for example, in the precocial sheep, unlike altricial species, the anatomical basis for visual depth perception is already established before birth.

Evidently some failures of adaptation are not corrected with the passage of time or further experience. Another example is that of individuals reared at altitude, of whom it has been reported that the carotid chemoreceptors are relatively inactive in later life. This raises the question of whether there might be other aspects of early development, perhaps uncorrected perinatally, which may have long-term effects upon the individual. In a study of which we shall hear more, David Barker, from the MRC Epidemiological Environmental Unit in Southampton, has gathered evidence which suggests that defective perinatal growth may be associated in adult life with the liability to hypertension and ischaemic heart disease. His work offers a stimulating challenge to all of us who are interested in the mechanisms by which fetuses adapt to their environment.

I look forward to our tackling this issue from a multidisciplinary point of view using the knowledge of traditional fetal physiology and endocrinology, supplemented by the skills of the molecular biologist and embryologist. I also wonder how our obstetric and neonatological colleagues will adapt to the problems which must arise from such an epidemiological surprise. If confirmed these observations will constitute a new stimulus to future research.

References

Basset JM, Bomford J, Mott JC (1988) Photoperiod: an important regulator of plasma prolactin concentration in fetal lambs during late gestation. Quart J Exp Physiol 73: 241–244.

Bocking AD, Harding R (1986) Effects of reduced uterine blood flow on electrocortical activity, breathing, and skeletal muscle activity in fetal sheep. Am J Obstet Gynecol 154: 655–662.

Bocking AD, Gagnon R, Milne KM, White SE (1988a) Behavioral activity during prolonged hypoxemia in fetal sheep. J Appl Physiol 65: 2420–2426.

Bocking AD, Gagnon R, White SE, Homan J, Milne KM, Richardson BS (1988b) Circulatory responses to prolonged hypoxaemia in fetal sheep. Am J Obstet Gynaecol 159: 1418–1424.

King AJ, Hutchings ME, Moore DR, Blakemore C (1988) Developmental plasticity in the visual and auditory representations in the mammalian superior colliculus. Nature 332: 73–76.

Kitanaka T, Alonso JG, Gilbert RD, Siu BL, Clemons GK, Longo LD (1989) Fetal responses to long-term hypoxaemia in sheep. Am J Physiol 256: R1340–1347.

Koos BJ, Kitanaka T, Matsuda K, Gilbert RD, Longo LD (1988) Fetal breathing adaptation to prolonged hypoxaemia in sheep. J Dev Physiol 10: 161–166.

Moore DR, Hutchings ME, King AJ, Kowalchuk NE (1989) The auditory brainstem of the ferret: effect of rearing with a unilateral ear plug on cochlear nucleus volume and projections to the inferior colliculus. J Neuroscience 9: 1213–1222.

Van der Loos (1977) Structural changes in the cerebral cortex upon modification of the periphery: barrels in the somato-sensory cortex. Philos Trans R Soc London B 278: 373–376.

Wiesel TN (1982) Postnatal development of the visual cortex and the influence of the environment. Nature 299: 583–591.

2

Fetal Baroreflexes and Chemoreflexes: Adaptation and Autonomy

M. HANSON

Department of Biochemistry and Physiology,
University of Reading, Reading, UK

It is highly appropriate to start a meeting concerned in part with 'fetal autonomy' by considering the reflexes elicited by baro- and chemoreceptors, as they are mediated almost entirely by the autonomic nervous system. Moreover, as the fetal mean arterial blood pressure and the mean arterial partial pressure of O_2 (p_aO_2) are different from those of the adult, it is important to discuss the extent to which these receptors operate in the fetal range of their adequate stimuli.

The term *adaptation* is often used to describe an organism which is well suited to its environment, in physiological and other ways. The term implies a degree of innate suitability to the environment, as opposed to the term *acclimatization*, which refers to the changes that the organism may undergo if its environment changes. In neurophysiology the term adaptation also has a more specific meaning, often applied to sensory receptors, namely the return of discharge towards control after a maintained change in the stimulus to the receptor. The degree of adaptation of the receptor is the extent to which its discharge returns towards its control level (even if that is zero, as for Pacinian corpuscles). Frequently the degree of adaptation depends on the *rate of change* of the stimulus. Moreover, the degree and rate of adaptation may depend on the *magnitude of the change* in stimulus and the baseline level from which the change occurs. The adaptive behaviour of the receptor is therefore hard to define, requiring continuous recording both of its afferent discharge and the stimulus to it.

Fetal Autonomy and Adaptation. Edited by G. S. Dawes, A. Zacutti, F. Borruto and A. Zacutti, Jr
© 1990 John Wiley & Sons Ltd

The Baroreflex

In the adult, adaptation has been well described for the arterial baroreceptors both on a short-term basis and over a longer period, e.g. in hypertension (see Sleight, 1980). This longer-term adaptation is often termed *resetting*. Fetal mean arterial pressure is lower in early rather than in late gestation, and pressure increases at birth when the low-resistance umbilical circulation is removed. We found in sheep that the carotid baroreceptors undergo resetting over the last third of gestation and the first postnatal month (Blanco et al., 1988). This resetting takes the form of a shift of the stimulus–response curve to a higher pressure range, such that basal discharge at the normal mean pressure does not change significantly, and also involves a reduction in the slope of the curve, so that the increase in discharge for any increase in pressure is reduced. From this information about the sensitivity of the afferents, it would be expected that baroreflexes can be elicited throughout this period, the *gain of the reflex loop* being reduced with gestational and postnatal age. Clinically, the interest in this area is in whether measurements of fetal heart rate can under any circumstances provide information about the operation of the baroreflex and the control of the circulation by the brainstem. A reflex fall in heart rate can indeed be produced in the sheep fetus by injecting a bolus of a vasoconstrictor such as phenylephrine i.v., and this change in heart rate is abolished by denervation of the baro- and chemoreceptors (Itskovitz et al., 1983). Apart from this, there is no agreement about the gain of the baroreflexes in the fetus in relation to that of the neonate or adult (see Hanson, 1989). These discrepancies may be due to differences in technique. A further complication is that, in the case of this reflex, the response (change in heart rate, cardiac output or peripheral resistance) changes the magnitude of the stimulus (arterial pressure) which has elicited it; thus there is a continuous interaction between stimulus and response, making the measurement of either difficult. The gain of the reflex needs to be measured under open-loop conditions, e.g. using isolated changes in pressure in the carotid sinus to elicit it, permitting the measurement of responses without interference from changes in the stimulus.

The operation of CNS processes which change the gain of the reflexes, and the balance between baro- and chemoreflexes, have to be included if adaptive mechanisms of the fetus as a whole are considered. Brainstem transection studies have provided some evidence for suprapontine processes affecting the gain of the baroreflex (Dawes et al., 1983) but at present we do not know their nature or location. The role of humoral agents has also to be considered as they may change during a trial or throughout development. For example, vasopressin is reported to affect the gain of the baroreflex (see Share, 1988, for review). We can only speculate about whether such processes play a role in controlling those aspects of fetal behaviour which differ from the neonate, and thus about the extent to which the fetus possesses processes which make it adapted to its environment.

Similar considerations also apply to reflexes elicited from the low-pressure side of the circulation, e.g. the response of the fetus to haemorrhage. Whilst its efferent limb involves the autonomic nervous system (Brace, 1987), it has been suggested that it depends more on chemo- than on baroreceptors for its afferent limb (Wood et al., 1989), unlike the adult. It is not known how this difference in balance is achieved.

The Arterial Chemoreflex

In both fetal sheep (Barcroft, 1946) and man (Soothill et al., 1986) at term p_aO_2 is about 25 mmHg, which is much lower than that of the adult. This raises the question of arterial chemoreceptor function in the fetus. Peripheral arterial chemoreceptor discharge is not maximal, as it would be in the adult at this p_aO_2, but is only about 5 Hz; it increases if p_aO_2 is reduced further (Blanco et al., 1984). Despite this increase in chemoreceptor afferent discharge in hypoxaemia or asphyxia, these stimuli do not produce an increase in breathing efforts (Boddy et al., 1974). Studies employing a range of techniques have failed to demonstrate chemoreflex effects on fetal breathing (see Hanson, 1990). In this respect, the fetus can be said to be adapted to its environment, as an increase in fetal breathing movements is wasteful of energy and does nothing for gas exchange. Again, knowledge about the function of CNS processes is crucial; in this case these processes operate to prevent an increase in chemoreceptor discharge from stimulating breathing movements (see Dawes, 1984). Future work must be aimed at determining the site and nature of these processes. The effects of hypoxia on breathing movements are abolished by transection of the brainstem through the upper pons (Dawes et al., 1983), or placement of lesions in the upper lateral pons (Gluckman and Johnston, 1987), but we do not know whether such techniques destroy a group of cells or pathways which mediate the response; nor do we know whether the neurones or tracts destroyed mediate the effect directly, or whether they provide a tonic input to the respiratory centres which determines the nature of the response. Recent work has shown that electrical stimulation of a more medial site in the pons can produce apnoea in the neonatal lamb (Coles et al., 1989) and that there are neurones in this area which are excited during hypoxia (Noble and Williams, 1989). We do not know whether or how this area is involved in the overall response of the fetus to hypoxia.

Whilst there are no chemoreflex effects on fetal breathing movements, such reflexes *do* exert effects on the fetal circulation under conditions of hypoxia or asphyxia, for example if uterine blood flow is reduced, and there is much clinical interest in studying the fetal circulation in an attempt to identify those fetuses which are not compensating adequately. The effect of hypoxia on the fetus at term is to produce a rapidly developing bradycardia, a more slowly developing increase in arterial blood pressure and a redistribution of cardiac output away from skeletal muscle and skin and towards the heart, brain, and adrenals. These effects are similar to those produced in adult animals by stimulating the arterial chemoreceptors while preventing the increase in ventilation which would normally occur (Daly and Scott, 1963). The chemoreflex nature of the effects in the fetus can be demonstrated by blocking the efferent limb or removing the afferent limb. The bradycardia is prevented by vagotomy or by atropine (see Martin, 1985) unless the asphyxia is intense and is maintained. The fall in heart rate is also delayed and attenuated by bilateral division of the carotid sinus nerves (Jensen and Hanson, 1989). The increase in arterial pressure is part of a complex redistribution of blood flow away from the carcass and towards the cerebral, coronary, and adrenal circulations (Rudolph, 1984). The extent to which this is reflex has yet to be determined and the complexity of the endocrine changes which also occur in hypoxia should not be underestimated (Hanson, 1989).

Responses to Hypoxia or Asphyxia

The intensity of a hypoxic or asphyxic challenge is one crucial aspect of it. A second aspect of the challenge is its *duration*. The effects of chronic hypoxia or reduction of placental function on fetal behaviour are only just beginning to be studied under experimental conditions in animals (Bocking et al., 1988a). Clearly a whole range of adaptive processes may be involved, including those in the periphery and in the CNS. It is interesting that fetal heart rate and blood pressure return to their pre-hypoxic levels over the first hour of hypoxia. Fetal breathing movements then also return after their initial cessation if the exposure to hypoxia is maintained for two or more days (Koos et al., 1988). In the neonatal kitten, chronic hypoxia appears to alter postnatal peripheral chemoreceptor resetting and results in a reduction in the sensitivity of the receptors to hypoxia (Hanson et al., 1989). We do not know the extent to which this represents adaptation of the receptors to hypoxia (a phenomenon which is not thought to occur in the adult) or whether it is some process which can be elicited only in the neonate, e.g. via an alteration in the degree or rate of postnatal chemoreceptor resetting. Whether or not a similar phenomenon occurs in the chronically hypoxic fetus is also not known, but it will clearly be of great clinical relevance to find out.

We know far less about the ability of the fetus to maintain circulatory redistribution during maintained hypoxia, e.g. to preserve cerebral blood flow (Richardson et al., 1989). In part this may depend on the degree of acidosis. In the absence of acidosis, it appears that fetal circulatory readjustments at 125–130 days gestation are maintained for 48 h after $p_a O_2$ is reduced from a mean of 23.4 to 17.3 mmHg by reduction of uterine blood flow (Bocking et al., 1988b).

A third aspect of a challenge is the *gestational age* at which it occurs. For example, hypoxia does not produce a significant bradycardia in fetal sheep between 97 and 102 days gestation (Boddy et al., 1974), unlike fetuses near term. This is probably not due to differences in peripheral chemoreceptor function: it may be due to differences in the CNS control mechanisms or at the effector level. Similarly, there are differences in the redistribution of blood flow during hypoxia in fetal sheep at 0.6–0.7 of term compared to that in term fetuses: in the younger fetuses, blood flow to muscle, skin, and gut does not fall (Iwamoto et al., 1989). As these authors speculate, this difference may be due to immaturity of arterial chemoreceptors, in the efferent limb of the reflex, or to differences in hormone (e.g. vasopressin) release.

Adaptation

In summary, the phenomenon of adaptation is pertinent to a variety of fetal systems at several levels of organization. To understand how it is operating under conditions where there is a challenge to fetal systems of control or autonomy, e.g. in asphyxia, it is necessary to have much more information about the components of the challenge that constitute a stimulus to the fetal receptors, and about the operation of the reflex loop at various gestational ages. To determine this we must have information gained simultaneously about both the stimuli and the responses. For each stimulus, we must know:

(a) its control level;
(b) its rate of change;
(c) the magnitude of its change;
(d) the duration of the change.

For each response, we need to know:

(a) how it relates to the stimulus parameters a–d above;
(b) whether it in turn changes the nature of the stimulus;
(c) how it interacts with other components of the overall response of the fetus.

These lists are somewhat daunting, and many of the items on them can only be found from the results of animal experiments, which then have to be extrapolated to man. But without knowledge of the processes of adaptation, it will not be possible to detect reliably those human fetuses which have not adapted adequately and hence which are at risk.

References

Barcroft J (1946) Researches on Pre-Natal Life. Blackwell Scientific Publications, Oxford.

Blanco CE, Dawes GS, Hanson MA, McCooke HB (1984) The response to hypoxia of arterial chemoreceptors in fetal sheep and new-born lambs, J Physiol 351: 25-37.

Blanco CE, Dawes GS, Hanson MA, McCooke HB (1988) Carotid baroreceptors in fetal and newborn sheep. Pediatr Res 24: 342-346.

Bocking AD, Gagnon R, Milne KM, White SE (1988a) Behavioral activity during prolonged hypoxemia in fetal sheep. J Appl Physiol 65: 2420-2426.

Bocking AD, Gagnon R, White SE, Homan J, Milne KM, Richardson BS (1988b) Circulatory responses to prolonged hypoxemia in fetal sheep. Am J Obstet Gynecol 159: 1418-1424.

Boddy K, Dawes GS, Fisher R, Pinter S, Robinson JS (1974) Foetal respiratory movements, electrocortical and cardiovascular responses to hypoxemia and hypercapnia in sheep. J Physiol 243: 599-618.

Brace RA (1987) Fetal blood volume responses to fetal haemorrhage: autonomic nervous system contribution. J Dev Physiol 9: 97-103.

Coles SK, Kumar P, Noble R (1989) Pontine sites inhibiting breathing in anaesthetized neonatal lambs. J Physiol 409: 66P.

Daly M de Burgh, Scott MJ (1963) The cardiovascular responses to stimulation of the carotid body chemoreceptors in the dog. J Physiol 165: 179-197.

Dawes GS (1984) The central control of fetal breathing and skeletal muscle movements. J Physiol 346: 1-18.

Dawes GS, Gardner WN, Johnston BM, Walker DW (1983) Breathing in fetal lambs: the effects of brain stem section. J Physiol 335: 535-553.

Gluckman PD, Johnston BM (1987) Lesions in the upper lateral pons abolish the hypoxic depression of breathing in unanaesthetized fetal lambs in utero. J Physiol 382: 373-383.

Hanson MA (1989) The importance of baro- and chemoreflexes in the control of the fetal cardiovascular system. J Dev Physiol 10: 491-511.

Hanson MA (1990) Peripheral control of fetal breathing. In: Fetal Physiology and Medicine (Eds: Johnston BM, Gluckman PD), pp. 191-204. Perinatology Press, Ithaca, New York.

Hanson MA, Eden GJ, Nijhuis JG, Moore PJ (1989) Peripheral chemoreceptors and other O_2 sensors in the fetus and newborn. In: Chemoreceptors and Reflexes in Breathing (Eds: Lahiri S, Forster RE, Davies RO, Pack AI), pp. 113-120. Oxford University Press, New York.

Itskovitz J, LaGamma EF, Rudolph AM (1983) Baroreflex control of the circulation in chronically instrumented fetal lambs. Circ Res 52: 589-596.

Iwamoto HS, Kaufman T, Keil LC, Rudolph AM (1989) Responses to acute hypoxemia in fetal sheep at 0.6-0.7 gestation. Am J Physiol 256: H613-H620.

Jensen A, Hanson MA (1989) Cardiovascular responses to acute asphyxia in carotid sinus denervated and intact fetal sheep near term. J Physiol 417: 19P.

Koos BJ, Kitanaka T, Matsuda K, Gilbert RD, Longo LD (1988) Fetal breathing adaptation to prolonged hypoxaemia in sheep. J Dev Physiol 10(2): 161-166.

Martin CB (1985) Pharmacological aspects of fetal heart rate regulation during hypoxia. In: Fetal Heart Rate Monitoring (Ed: Kunzel W), pp. 170-184. Springer-Verlag, Berlin.

Noble R, Williams BA (1989) Excitation of neurones in the rostral pons during hypoxia in anaesthetized neonatal lambs. J Physiol 417: 146P.

Richardson BS, Rurak DW, Patrick JE, Homan J, Carmichael L (1989) Cerebral oxidative metabolism during sustained hypoxaemia in fetal sheep. J Dev Physiol 11: 37-43.

Rudolph AM (1984) The fetal circulation and its response to stress. J Dev Physiol 6: 11-19.

Share L (1988) Role of vasopressin in cardiovascular regulation. Physiol Rev 68: 1248–1284.

Sleight P (1980) Arterial Baroreceptors and Hypertension. Oxford University Press, Oxford.

Soothill, PW, Nicolaides KH, Rodeck CH, Campbell S (1986) Effect of gestational age on fetal and intervillous blood gas and acid-base values in human pregnancy. Fetal Therapy 1: 168–175.

Wood CE, Chen H-G, Bell ME (1989) Role of vagosympathetic fibers in the control of adrenocorticotropic hormone, vasopressin, and renin responses to hemorrhage in fetal sheep. Circ Res 64: 515–523.

Discussion

The Baroreflex

Thornburg asked whether the change in slope of the baroreflex with postnatal age was a consequence of the perinatal rise in arterial pressure, or whether it was genetically programmed. [Reference to Dr Thornburg's paper will show the dramatic changes in ventricular function curves which take place at birth, after ventilation of the lungs: ed.] Would the change in slope still occur if arterial pressure did not alter at birth? Hanson did not know the answer; he regarded it as an important question and had considered it. There were difficulties in designing experiments to cause a chronic reduction or elevation in arterial pressure in the fetus in utero, to test the point.

Several possible mechanisms of adaptation by the baroreflex were considered by Ellendorff and Hanson. They included local changes (viscoelastic) in the vessel(s), at the cellular level in the baroreceptor, in afferent axons, possible gating or change in gain in the central nervous system, and in efferent pathways. None had been systematically studied.

Systemic Arterial Chemoreceptors

John Patrick then raised the question of the adaptation of systemic chemoreceptors in the carotid and the aortic arch. Hanson had shown, by direct single fibre recording in sheep, that their adaptation was slow, over days or weeks, compared with that of the baroreceptors, some components of which adapt within an hour or so. Patrick quoted the work of Bocking et al. (1988a,b), who had shown that prolonged isocapnic hypoxia (a 40–50% reduction in O_2 content) caused only transient changes in fetal heart rate and arterial pressure in unanaesthetized sheep in utero, but a more prolonged reduction in fetal breathing and body movements. However within 8–10 hours they too had returned to normal in spite of continued hypoxaemia. He speculated that the

adaptation was too rapid to be cellular. Total cerebral blood flow was increased
and O_2 uptake was maintained at normal levels. Coronary blood flow was
greatly increased, with almost total O_2 extraction. Adaptation was too rapid
to be due to an increase in haemoglobin concentration. There was no evidence
of a gross change in the oxyhaemoglobin dissociation curve.

The possibility of concurrent hormonal changes was considered. Plasma
catecholamines were known to rise greatly during fetal hypoxia, near term; the
effect is dependent on gestational age. However, during prolonged hypoxia they
return to near the initial value after a few hours. John Challis reported that
the same was true of fetal plasma ACTH and cortisol; however, after 18–24
hours the plasma cortisol concentration started to rise again, as if the pituitary-
adrenal axis had been chronically activated (Challis et al., 1989). Little was
known about long-term changes in fetal plasma vasopressin, though there is
a four-fold initial rise at the onset of hypoxia, which could in part explain the
rise in arterial pressure. Some of these hormonal changes might be of clinical
interest as indicating prolonged hypoxia, e.g. erythropoietin.

Adaptation to Alcohol

John Patrick mentioned the fetal response to maternal alcohol ingestion, as
another puzzling instance of adaptation. On first administration breathing
movements of fetal lambs in utero are arrested. But after a few days fetal
behaviour returns to normal in spite of chronic alcohol administration. There
is, during this time, no change in the distribution or rate of elimination of alcohol
in mother or fetus; there is no evidence of enzyme induction in the fetal liver
(Clarke et al., 1988; Smith et al., 1989).

In chronic alcoholic human mothers also it had been reported that the patterns
of fetal behaviour, including breathing movements, were normal. The
mechanisms of tolerance or adaptation were not known.

Hanson also mentioned the strange responses to administration of a
prostaglandin synthetase inhibitor, meclofenamate, which caused continuous
fetal breathing movements in sheep after a delay of 30–40 minutes, lasting several
hours (Wallen et al., 1988). The possibility of gradual adaptation to the changes
observed should be considered.

Chronic Hypoxaemia and Brain Damage

Finally Ellendorff started a discussion on the long-term effects of hypoxaemia
on the central nervous system (continued subsequently in Chapters 13 and 14).
He referred to the likelihood of critical periods in the CNS response, and drew
attention to the fact that brief hypoxia at birth could cause hippocampal damage

and epilepsy in adults. However, the immediate discussion made it evident that, while there was evidence of brain damage on short-term exposure of fetal animals to severe hypoxia, long-term exposure to mild or moderate hypoxia (such as might occur prenatally in growth-retarded human fetuses) had not been explored systematically. So we do not know whether this might cause irreversible or total recovery; the plasticity of the CNS in early development, established in other experimental work, has to be considered. It is difficult to do properly controlled experiments, with repeated measurements of the blood gases, in fetuses of small inexpensive laboratory animals.

References

Bocking AD, Gagnon R, Milne KM, White SE (1988a) J Appl Physiol 65: 2420.
Bocking AD, Gagnon R, White SE, Homan J, Milne KM, Richardson BS (1988b) Am J Obstet Gynecol 159: 1418.
Challis JRG, Fraher L, Oosterhuis J, White SE, Bocking AD (1989) Am J Obstet Gynecol 160: 926–932.
Clarke DW, Smith GN, Patrick J et al. (1988) Drug Met Dispos 16: 464–468.
Smith GN, Brien JF, Carmichael L et al. (1989) J Dev Physiol 11: 189–197.
Wallen LD, Murai DT, Clyman RI, Lee CH, Mauray FE, Kitterman JA (1988) J Appl Physiol 64: 759–766.

3

Fetal Cardiac Output and its Distribution

K. L. THORNBURG, M. J. MORTON, C. W. PINSON,
M. D. RELLER, G. D. GIRAUD AND D. L. REID

School of Medicine, Oregon Health Sciences University, Portland, Oregon, USA

Much of what we know about the function of the fetal heart and the distribution of its output has been learned during the last two decades. The past 10 years have been particularly fruitful for new findings in the fetus because of extensive pioneer work by first-rate investigators in the fields of ventricular and circulatory function in adult animals. But it was not until the 1970s that the techniques of earlier adult work could be appropriately adapted to the conscious fetal mammal. Therefore, our present knowledge of fetal haemodynamics and cardiac function only now begins to compare with the level of knowledge of adult cardiovascular physiology in the late 1960s.

In addition to recent technological advances in fetal physiology, new molecular techniques have become available for studying the fetal heart. These advances, while not ends in themselves, provide access to another level of investigation in the search for the mechanisms that underlie the physiological behaviour of the fetus. With the new in mind, the purpose of this chapter is to discuss recent advances in cardiac physiology, to highlight current controversies, and to indicate fertile directions for research in the future.

Ventricular Function

Until recently it was generally believed by fetal experts that the ventricles of the fetal heart were anatomically and physiologically similar (Dawes, 1968; St John Sutton et al., 1984). However, recent work indicates that the right and left ventricles, while more similar in fetal life than in adult life, are distinctly

Fetal Autonomy and Adaptation. Edited by G. S. Dawes, A. Zacutti, F. Borruto and A. Zacutti, Jr
©1990 John Wiley & Sons Ltd

different during prenatal development. In a study of late gestation fetal sheep hearts we found that the right ventricle has a thinner wall, a greater radius of curvature and a greater chamber volume at any positive transmural filling pressure than does the left ventricle (Table 1) (Pinson et al., 1987). These findings lead one to predict that the ventricles will have different physiological behaviours also. Such a prediction can be made on the basis of Laplace's law when simplistically applied to the equatorial plane of the ventricular free wall. Laplace's law states that the stress in the wall of a thin-walled sphere (S_w) is equal to one half the transmural pressure across the wall of the sphere (P_t) times the ratio of the radius of curvature (r) to the wall thickness (h):

$$S_w = P_t/2 \cdot r/h$$

At any given transmural pressure, it is clear that wall tension depends on the radius to wall-thickness ratio. Therefore, even at similar transmural pressures, as during fetal life (Thornburg and Morton, 1986), wall stress must be higher in the ventricle with the largest radius to thickness ratio—the right ventricle.

Current evidence demonstrates that the ventricles behave differently from one another as predicted. The right ventricle ejects a larger stroke volume than the left ventricle at common filling and arterial pressures (Heymann et al., 1973; Anderson et al., 1981) thus demonstrating fetal right ventricular dominance. Furthermore, right ventricular stroke volume is more easily depressed by increases in arterial pressure than is left stroke volume, either under normoxic (Thornburg and Morton, 1986; Reller et al., 1987) or hypoxaemic conditions (Reller et al., 1989). It should be noted, however, that the issue of arterial pressure sensitivity is controversial and requires further study (Hawkins et al., 1989). Studies on the form of the fetal heart indicate that the right ventricle develops into the larger chamber of the two ventricles but only at the expense of decreased right ventricular function under systolic pressure loading conditions.

TABLE 1   Cardiac weights and other parameters in the sheep fetus

	$(n = 44)$
Fetal weight (kg)	2.9 ± 0.8
Ventricular weight (g)	16.0 ± 4.8
RV/LV free wall weight	0.94 ± 0.14
	$(n = 10)$
RV free wall thickness (mm)	3.0 ± 0.7
LV free wall thickness (mm)	4.2 ± 0.7
RV radius/thickness ratio (r/h)	4.5 ± 0.9
LV radius/thickness ratio (r/h)	2.6 ± 0.9
RV volume (ml)	5.6 ± 1.4
LV volume (ml)	4.2 ± 1.6

Cardiac Adaptations at Birth

It has long been known that cardiac output is augmented at birth and that the stroke volumes of the two ventricles equalize during the postnatal transition period (Figure 1). Cross-sectional data indicate that the stroke volumes of both ventricles increase at birth and that left ventricular stroke volume must increase by nearly two times to equal the 30% postnatal increase in right ventricular stroke volume (Klopfenstein and Rudolph, 1978; Lister et al., 1979; Anderson et al., 1981). Cardiac output can increase by any of several known mechanisms: increased heart rate, increased preload, decreased afterload, increased contractility, or enlargement of the cardiac chamber. In the early neonatal period, heart rate increases significantly from about 170 to over 200 beats/minute (Berman and Musselman, 1979) but this does not explain stroke volume increases. Other mechanisms must be at work.

As the fetal circulation is transformed into its neonatal form, with pulmonary and systemic circuits pumping in series (Rudolph and Heymann, 1973), loading conditions for both ventricles are dramatically altered. Left ventricular filling pressure becomes greater than right ventricular filling pressure, creating a significant diastolic pressure 'gradient' across the cardiac septum (Figure 2). Arterial pressure in the systemic circuit increases by 20–30 mmHg, augmenting left ventricular afterload, while decreased pressure in the pulmonary circuit (20–30 mmHg) reduces afterload for the right ventricle (Figure 3). Contractility is significantly augmented during the transition period (Riemenschnieder et al, 1981; Anderson et al., 1984), which may in part be due to increased levels of circulating catecholamines. The modest increase in right ventricular stroke

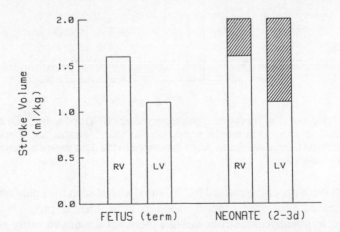

FIGURE 1   Estimates of right (RV) and left ventricular (LV) stroke volumes in the prenatal (fetus) and the immediate postnatal (neonate) periods of lambs. Hatched portion is SV (stroke volume) increase after birth, estimated from cross-sectional data

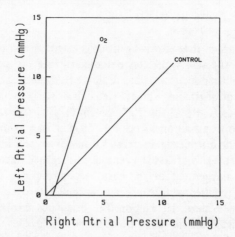

FIGURE 2   Mean left atrial pressure versus right atrial pressure in fetal sheep before (control) and after 30 minutes of in utero ventilation with 100% oxygen (O_2). Note that left atrial pressure is about three times higher than right atrial pressure during O_2 ventilation. Revised from Morton et al. (1987)

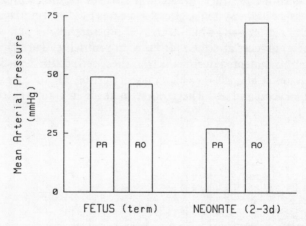

FIGURE 3   Estimates of pressures in pulmonary artery (PA) and aorta (AO) before and after birth. The disparity in arterial pressures after birth indicates that afterload in the left ventricle (AO) increases dramatically compared to the right ventricle. From idealized cross-sectional data

volume at birth may be explained by decreased afterload in the pulmonary circuit and increased inotropic support (though experimental proof is lacking). However, left ventricular stroke volume increases are not so easily explained. Left ventricular stroke volume rises dramatically at birth, even though the left ventricle must eject its stroke volume against a higher arterial pressure. Furthermore, left ventricular output is increased in newborn lambs *even after*

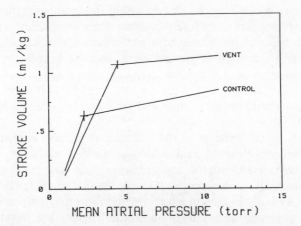

FIGURE 4   Left ventricular (LV) function curves in eight fetal sheep near term. LV stroke volume was measured by electromagnetic flow probe and is plotted versus mean left atrial pressure before (control) and after in utero ventilation with oxygen (vent). Curves are made by rapidly withdrawing and reinfusing blood. Augmentation of stroke volume at birth has not been satisfactorily explained since changes in preload or afterload alone do not bring about such large increases

beta-adrenergic receptors have been antagonized (Klopfenstein and Rudolph, 1978). We have shown that the ventilation of fetuses with oxygen while in utero decreases their pulmonary vascular resistance to nearly newborn levels (Reid and Thornburg, 1987) and that a trans-septal pressure gradient is established (Thornburg and Morton, 1986; Morton et al., 1987). This causes an upward shift in the left ventricular function curve, which means that stroke volume increases to neonatal levels at all physiological filling pressures. The upward shift of the function curve occurs even in the presence of propranolol, which blocks the beta-adrenergic stimulating effects of catecholamines (Figure 4). However, the mechanisms behind the increase in stroke volume at birth have not yet been satisfactorily explained. Several possibilities should be explored. For example, Breall et al. (1984) suggest that thyroid hormone may play an important role in the augmentation of stroke volume. Because the natal increase in left ventricular stroke volume rises in concert with the establishment of a left-right pressure gradient, we favour a mechanical explanation for the change in left ventricular stroke volume at birth. But the real explanation of this important adaptation at birth awaits further research.

Cardiac Growth

The fetal myocardium is well suited for growth regulation studies because the fetal heart grows rapidly and because both haemodynamic and humoral aspects of the regulatory process can be altered within the uterine environment. The cardiac myocyte appears to mature through a series of genetically determined patterns, each being characteristic of a particular stage of development. For example, early in embryonic development, myocytes grow by both cell enlargement (hypertrophy) and by cell division (hyperplasia). In fetal life, cells grow only by hyperplasia, maintaining a constant cell size. However, soon after birth, cardiac myocytes stop dividing and grow forever after by hypertrophy alone (Oparil, 1985).

Another interesting feature of the maturation process is that immature myocytes are mononuclear but tend to become binuclear as they mature (Clubb and Bishop, 1984). Furthermore, adult cells are commonly polyploid, though there is great variation among species (Oparil, 1985). Though the heart appears to go through a change in growth modes (hyperplastic to hypertrophic growth) at a critical postnatal stage, it is uncertain whether the development of binucleation and polyploidy is directly related to these changes in mode. The nature of the 'switch' that turns off the hyperplastic growth mode after birth is also not known.

In our laboratory we are investigating growth regulation in fetal sheep under conditions of pressure overload. We are administering a systolic pressure load to each heart ventricle separately for a period of 10 days by placing an inflatable occluder around the appropriate artery, adding a 10–15 mmHg mean pressure load to each ventricle. Pressure loading the right ventricle causes it to grow more rapidly than normal (Pinson et al., 1985). This growth alters the functional capability of the ventricle as predicted by Laplace's law. The loaded right ventricle becomes 'stronger' and more resistant to increases in arterial pressure (Pinson et al., 1985). (A similar phenomenon was seen by Alonso et al. (1989) in fetuses subjected to prolonged hypoxaemia). Our preliminary data indicate that myocytes do not grow by hypertrophy alone when pressure loaded during fetal life, but rather, most growth is hyperplastic under these conditions. This finding was predicted by the study of Fishman et al. (1978). From these studies and those of Momma and Takoa (1989), one can hypothesize that the small ventricle in the fetal 'hypoplastic syndrome' is actually the result of a hyperplastic growth response to loading that eventually obliterates the ventricular chamber. This hypothesis needs to be tested in an experimental model by use of cytomorphometric techniques. Our preliminary findings suggest that pressure loading tends to speed up myocyte maturation as indicated by the portion of cells that are binuclear. In our preliminary experiments, loaded hearts tend to have increased numbers of binuclear myocytes compared to unloaded control hearts. More experiments are required before this is known for certain.

Several other growth-related problems badly need investigative attention. In addition to the role of mechanical loading in affecting growth of the myocyte, there is a great need to identify the primary humoral regulators of myocyte growth in the fetal and neonatal period. Although growth factors have been investigated in the fetus, little attention has been paid to their role in myocyte growth. Whether, for example, polypeptide growth factors behave specifically as 'competence' factors (King et al., 1989), affecting the G_1 portion of the cell cycle, or as 'progression' factors, promoting progression through other portions of the cell cycle, is not known. We also need to understand the regulation of growth of non-myocyte cells if we are to understand the general phenomenon known as 'ventricular remodelling'. The regulation of fibroblast growth and its role in determining the architecture of the fetal heart is a crucial piece of the growth puzzle, yet it has not been investigated.

Lastly, the regulation of capillary density in the growing fetus is a crucial problem because it is likely that prenatal blood vessel growth determines the distribution of blood in the adult myocardium.

Distribution of Cardiac Output

The most powerful tool in studying blood flow distribution in the fetus has been the radiolabelled microsphere technique (Heymann et al., 1977). This technique enables the quantification of blood flow and changes in flow distribution under various physiological and pathophysiological conditions. Acute fetal hypoxaemia has been the most widely studied (Cohn et al., 1974; Sheldon et al., 1979; Ashwal et al., 1980; Reuss and Rudolph, 1980; Reller et al., 1989) but flow distribution has also been investigated under conditions of haemorrhage (Itskovitz et al., 1982), umbilical flow restriction (Itskovitz, et al., 1987), and during the infusion of various vasoactive substances. Rudolph (1984) reviewed the redistribution of arterial oxygen delivery to fetal organs under conditions of hypoxaemia (maternal hypoxia) and umbilical cord compression. The message from these studies is that oxygen delivery (blood flow × oxygen content) to fetal heart, brain, and adrenal glands is dramatically increased under hypoxaemic conditions; myocardial oxygen delivery actually doubles. However, when the umbilical cord is compressed, oxygen delivery to brain and heart is little changed even with a reduction of umbilical flow by 50%. In both kinds of stress, oxygen delivery to other organs is reduced.

The mechanisms that underlie the response to acute hypoxaemia are not well studied, though it is well known that the baroreceptor mechanism responds to the usual increase in arterial pressure that accompanies the acute phase. Rudolph believes that the chemoreceptors are also critical in determining the fetal response (Rudolph, 1984). The typical bradycardic response to hypoxaemia is abolished with autonomic blockade (Iwamoto et al., 1983) but blood flow is still redistributed to maintain oxygenation of heart and brain. Studies from our laboratory indicate that the reduction of cardiac output with hypoxaemia can be explained by increased afterload which directly affects stroke volume, particularly of the right ventricle (Reller et al., 1989).

TABLE 2   Blood flow to fetal organs during in utero
ventilation with oxygen

Organ	Teitel (1988)	Blanco et al. (1988)
	(percent change in flow)	
Lung	+554	—
Heart	−65	−40
Brain	−62	−70
Placenta	−36	−67
Kidney	−38	−24

Cardiac Output Distribution at Birth

The advent of the in utero ventilation technique (Faber et al., 1979) has allowed
the birth process to be studied in stages. Two particularly good studies have
determined the distribution of near term fetal cardiac output with microspheres,
while ventilating the fetal lungs with an oxygen-rich mixture (Blanco et al., 1988;
Teitel, 1988). Both demonstrated the major changes in blood flow to various
organs during the establishment of the neonatal circulation. The Teitel study
also emphasized changes during ventilation and cord occlusion while the Blanco
study gave emphasis to the levels of oxygenation. Table 2 shows the changes
in distribution of flow during in utero oxygenation. Perhaps the most interesting
and novel finding is that placental flow is greatly reduced with in utero ventilation
and is clearly dependent on oxygen partial pressure. The redistribution of blood
volume during the transition period has not been studied, but one could
hypothesize that placental blood volume is decreased as pulmonary volume is
greatly expanded.

The Calcium Cycle and Cardiac Function

Within the myocyte the cycle of tension generation and relaxation is determined
by the myoplasmic calcium concentration—$[Ca^{2+}]$—(Fabiato and Fabiato,
1978). However, the $[Ca^{2+}]$ in the cell is in turn regulated by specialized
membrane proteins of the muscle cell membrane (sarcolemma) and the
sarcoplasmic reticulum. The slow inward current of the action potential is
primarily carried by calcium ions from extracellular fluid moving through two
populations of channels in the sarcolemma (Bean, 1985). This calcium is thought
to trigger the required release of calcium from the sarcoplasmic reticulum that
activates the contractile apparatus at each contraction. Relaxation of tension
is caused by the removal of myoplasmic calcium by the Na–Ca exchange protein
in the cell membrane, by the ATPase on the sarcoplasmic reticulum and perhaps
by an ATPase on the sarcolemma (of unknown importance) (Carafoli and

Zurini, 1982). As calcium is pumped from the myoplasm, and $[Ca^{2+}]$ falls, the contractile proteins are 'deactivated' and tension falls.

In the developing heart it is important to know the relative rate of maturation of each of these membrane-bound proteins, because they determine myocyte function and ultimately cardiac function. There is considerable variation among species as to the relative stage of development when sarcoplasmic reticulum and transverse tubules develop. T-tubules do not develop until after birth in rat, mouse, rabbit, dog, and hamster but develop before birth in monkey, cow, guinea pig, and sheep (reviewed by Smolich, 1987). But how does the cell relax and contract before the sarcoplasmic reticulum is mature? Recent evidence indicates that the sarcolemma is responsible for regulating intracellular calcium stores before the sarcoplasmic reticulum becomes mature (Klitzner and Friedman, 1989), but further work is needed to understand this aspect of cardiac electrophysiology.

The correlation of the development of cardiac function and the maturation of the biochemical and electrophysiological components of growing myocytes has not been well studied. Little is known of whether the calcium-binding proteins develop concomitantly with the contractile proteins; their molecular regulation is a field of study that beckons the eager molecular biologist.

Summary

The purpose of this article has been to focus on several areas of fetal cardiac research that are ripe for progress. The primary areas covered include fetal ventricular function, cardiac adaptations at birth, cardiac growth, the myocyte calcium cycle, and regulation of the distribution of cardiac output. Each of these areas needs to be approached with fresh new ways of thinking with a clear avoidance of the idea that fetal physiology will mimic adult physiology on a small scale. Since the 1960s fetal physiologists have been demonstrating that the fetal heart is not merely a miniature adult heart, either in form or in function. Dawes' 1968 monograph, *Foetal and Neonatal Physiology*, was instrumental in indicating to the scientific world the many ways in which the fetus is physiologically unique. Even so, the miniature adult notion, like the homunculus notion before it, has not been easily dispelled and continues to hamper clear thinking by those inside and outside the field. Lastly, our scientific colleagues and funding agencies alike need to be reminded that knowledge of the developing organism is the foundation for understanding the mature organism. Explorations into the world of the unborn will bring benefit to young and old alike.

Acknowledgements

The authors offer heartfelt thanks to Jackie Niemi and Jean Matsumoto for secretarial support. Tom Green, Robert Webber, Pat Renwick, Karen Lentfer,

Sharon Kinney, Sharon Gasser, Nick Schiller, Paul Klas, Alisa Eicher, and Marilyn Paul provided superb technical help.

This work was supported by grants from the National Institutes of Health (HD10034, HL43015), from the American Heart Association, Oregon Affiliate, and from the Medical Research Foundation of Oregon.

References

Alonso JG, Okai T, Longo LD, Gilbert RD (1989) Cardiac function during long-term hypoxemia in fetal sheep. Am J Physiol 257: H581–H589.

Anderson DF, Bissonnette JM, Faber JJ, Thornburg KL (1981) Central shunt flows and pressures in the mature fetal lamb. Am J Physiol 241: H60–H66.

Anderson PAW, Glick KL, Manring A, Crenshaw C Jr (1984) Developmental changes in cardiac contractility in fetal and postnatal sheep: in vitro and in vivo. Am J Physiol 247: H371–H379.

Ashwal S, Majcher JS, Vain N, Longo LD (1980) Patterns of fetal lamb regional cerebral blood flow during and after prolonged hypoxia. Pediatr Res 14: 1104–1110.

Bean BP (1985) Two kinds of calcium channels in canine atrial cells. J Gen Physiol 86: 1–30.

Berman W Jr, Musselman J (1979) Myocardial performance in the newborn lamb. Am J Physiol 237: H66–H70.

Blanco CE, Martin CB, Rankin J, Landauer M, Phernetton T (1988) Changes in fetal organ flow during intrauterine mechanical ventilation with or without oxygen. J Develop Physiol 10: 53–62.

Breall JA, Rudolph AM, Heymann MA (1984) Role of thyroid hormone in postnatal circulatory and metabolic adjustments. J Clin Invest 73: 1418–1424.

Carafoli E, Zurini M (1982) The Ca^{2+}-pumping ATPase of plasma membranes: purification, reconstitution and properties. Biochim Biophys Acta 683: 279–301.

Clubb FJ Jr, Bishop SP (1984) Formation of binucleated myocardial cells in the neonatal rat: an index for growth hypertrophy. Lab Invest 50: 571–577.

Cohn HE, Sacks EJ, Heymann MA, Rudolph AM (1974) Cardiovascular responses to hypoxemia and acidemia in fetal lambs. Am J Obstet Gynecol 120: 817–824.

Dawes GS (1968) Foetal and Neonatal Physiology: A Comparative Study of the Changes at Birth. Year Book Medical Publishers, Chicago.

Faber JJ, Bissonnette JM, Thornburg KL (1979) In utero ventilation of the unanesthetized near term lamb. Physiologist 22: 4.

Fabiato A, Fabiato F (1978) Calcium-induced release of calcium from the sarcoplasmic reticulum of skinned cells from adult human, dog, cat, rabbit, rat and frog hearts and from fetal and new-born rat ventricles. Ann NY Acad Sci 307: 491–522.

Fishman NH, Hof RB, Rudolph AM, Heymann MA (1978) Models of congenital heart disease in fetal lambs. Circulation 58: 354–364.

Hawkins J, Van Hare GF, Schmidt KG, Rudolph AM (1989) Effects of increasing afterload on left ventricular output in fetal lambs. Circ Res 65: 127–134.

Heymann MA, Creasy RK, Rudolph AM (1973) Quantitation of blood flow pattern in the foetal lamb in utero. In: Foetal and Neonatal Physiology, Proceedings of the Sir Joseph Barcroft Centenary Symposium (Eds: Comline KS, Cross KW, Dawes GS, Nathanielsz PW) pp. 129–135. Cambridge University Press, Cambridge.

Heymann MA, Payne BD, Hoffman JIE, Rudolph AM (1977) Blood flow measurements with radionuclide labeled microspheres. Prog Cardiovasc Dis 20: 55–77.

Itskovitz J, Goetzman BW, Rudolph AM (1982) Effects of hemorrhage on umbilical venous return and oxygen delivery in fetal lambs. Am J Physiol 242: H543–H548.

Itskovitz J, LaGamma EF, Rudolph AM (1987) Effects of cord compression on fetal blood flow distribution and O_2 delivery. Am J Physiol 252: H100–H109.

Iwamoto HS, Rudolph AM, Mirkin BL, Keil LC (1983) Circulatory and humoral responses of sympathectomized fetal sheep to hypoxemia. Am J Physiol 245: H767–H772.

King RJ, Jones MB, Minoo P (1989) Regulation of lung cell proliferation by polypeptide growth factors. Am J Physiol 257: L23–L38.

Klitzner TS, Friedman WF (1989) A diminished role for the sarcoplasmic reticulum in newborn myocardial contraction: effects of ryanodine. Pediatr Res 26: 98–101.

Klopfenstein HS, Rudolph AM (1978) Postnatal changes in the circulation and responses to volume loading in sheep. Circ Res 42: 839–845.

Lister G, Walter TK, Versmold HT, Dallman PT, Rudolph AM (1979) Oxygen delivery in lambs: cardiovascular and hematologic development. Am J Physiol 237: H668–H675.

Momma K, Takao A (1989) Right ventricular concentric hypertrophy and left ventricular dilatation by ductal constriction in fetal rats. Circ Res 64: 1137–1146.

Morton MJ, Pinson CW, Thornburg KL (1987) In utero ventilation with oxygen augments left ventricular stroke volume in lambs. J Physiol 383: 413–424.

Oparil S (1985) Morphologic substrates of sudden death: pathogenesis of ventricular hypertrophy. J Am Coll Cardiol 5: 57B–65B.

Pinson CW, Morton MJ, Thornburg KL (1985) Fetal right ventricular adaptation to chronic pressure overload. Fed Proc 44: 466.

Pinson CW, Morton MJ, Thornburg KL (1987) An anatomic basis for fetal right ventricular dominance and arterial pressure sensitivity. J Develop Physiol 9: 253–269.

Reid DL, Thornburg KL (1987) Pulmonary vascular resistance (PVR) of conscious fetal lambs during in utero ventilation. Physiologist 30: 183.

Reller MD, Morton MJ, Reid DL, Thornburg KL (1987) Fetal lamb ventricles respond differently to filling and arterial pressures and to in utero ventilation. Pediatr Res 22: 621–626.

Reller MD, Morton MJ, Giraud GD, Reid DL, Thornburg KL (1989) The effect of acute hypoxemia on ventricular function during β-adrenergic and cholinergic blockade in the fetal lamb. J Develop Physiol 11: 263–269.

Reuss ML, Rudolph AM (1980) Distribution and recirculation of umbilical and systemic venous blood flow in fetal lambs during hypoxia. J Develop Physiol 2: 71–84.

Riemenschneider TA, Brenner RA, Mason DT (1981) Maturational changes in myocardial contractile state of newborn lambs. Pediatr Res 15: 349–356.

Rudolph AM (1984) The fetal circulation and its response to stress. J Develop Physiol 6: 11–19.

Rudolph AM, Heymann MA (1973) Control of the foetal circulation. In: Foetal and Neonatal Physiology: Proceedings of the Sir Joseph Barcroft Centenary Symposium (Eds: Comline KS, Cross KW, Dawes GS, Nathanielsz PW) pp 89–111. Cambridge University Press, Cambridge.

Sheldon RE, Peeters LLH, Makowski EL, Meschia G (1979) Redistribution of cardiac output and oxygen delivery in the hypoxemic fetal lamb. Am J Obstet Gynecol 135: 1071–1078.

Smolich J (1987) Morphology of the developing myocardium. In: Perinatal Development of the Heart and Lung (Eds: Lipshitz J, Maloney J, Nimrod C, Carson G). Perinatology Press, Ithaca, NY.

St John Sutton MG, Raichlen JS, Reichek N, Huff DS (1984) Quantitative assessment of right and left ventricular growth in the human fetal heart: a pathoanatomic study. Circulation 70: 935–941.

Teitel DF (1988) Circulatory adjustments to postnatal life. Sem Perinatol 12: 96–103.

Thornburg KL, Morton MJ (1986) Filling and arterial pressures as determinants of left ventricular stroke volume in fetal lambs. Am J Physiol 251: H961–H968.

Discussion

Ventricular Size and Hyperplasia

In response to questions from Patrick, Thornburg explained that in fetal lambs the right ventricle is larger and has a larger stroke volume, but because of its size it has a greater radius/wall thickness ratio and so it is at a mechanical disadvantage. The fetus has a small round left ventricle, well suited to generating a high pressure after birth. The larger weaker right ventricle is not so well endowed. Consequently infants with transposition of the great arteries are at a disadvantage postnatally.

Thornburg also speculated about the consequences of valvular and other anomalies causing an increased resistance in a ventricular outflow tract. As a consequence of the increased pressure the wall would grow thicker, obliterating its own chamber, a process that was hyperplastic, not hypoplastic as convention has hitherto dictated.

Pardi raised the question of ventricular size and adaptation in human infants, with increasing gestational age or intrauterine growth retardation. Thornburg said that more factual information was needed. Sahn et al. (1980) and Wladimiroff and McGhie (1980) had shown that ventricular sizes and stroke volumes were not identical as previously supposed; right ventricular output was greater in normal fetuses. In the subsequent discussion it became evident that the findings of Reed et al. (1987), who had reported an increased ratio of the right:left ventricular flow in growth retardation (2.1:1 as compared with 1.3:1 in normal fetuses), was controversial on the grounds of case selection and for other reasons. There was agreement with Thornburg's suggestion that the manufacturers of ultrasound equipment should be encouraged to produce instruments to measure blood vessel or cardiac orifice diameter *simultaneously* with mean blood flow velocity. There were evident pitfalls in calculations of blood flow (ml/min) derived from estimates of velocity and diameter made at different times.

Oxygen Delivery and Coronary Flow

Pardi then asked whether the relative low oxygen availability in human fetuses with growth retardation and chronic compensated hypoxaemia, might alter ventricular function. Thornburg thought this unlikely because of the astonishing ability of the coronary circulation to dilate and hence maintain oxygen supply to the heart. In well-oxygenated fetuses O_2 extraction in the coronary vasculature was almost complete, so that the pO_2 in coronary sinus blood was only 4–7 mmHg. In fetal lambs made acutely hypoxic (by maternal ventilation with low O_2 mixtures) there was a large increase in coronary blood flow (Fisher et al., 1982), and ventricular function, measured directly in utero, was maintained (Reller et al., 1989). Oxygen delivery kept up with demand. Ultimately, however, the ventricles, especially the right ventricle, became sensitive to changes in arterial pressure. Since a possible inference was that fetal hydrops might not then be a consequence of heart failure, Dawes drew attention to the hydrops seen in terminal human fetal tachyarrhythmias, in rhesus incompatibility and in the gross hypertension induced by Mott in fetal lambs. Thornburg thought that there might be explanations for these phenomena other than volume overload. However, there are differences between the results of acute and chronic hypoxaemia, and growth retardation has other effects on fetal protein metabolism (Chapter 11). There was as yet no direct or indirect evidence of changes in arterial pressure in growth retardation in human infants.

The mechanisms of blood flow redistribution to heart and brain in hypoxaemia were discussed. Thornburg said that autonomic blockade did not greatly alter the redistribution (Iwamoto et al., 1983). Patrick commented on the remarkable degree of autoregulation in these organs, in which O_2 delivery and metabolism continued to be well matched under extreme conditions, in contrast to most other organs. The mechanisms, presumably locally mediated vasodilatation in response to reduced pO_2 and elevated pCO_2, required study.

Control of Cardiac Ventricular Growth

Thornburg said that the ventricles responded to hypertension induced by partial occlusion of the descending aorta above the origin of the renal arteries, by a rapid increase in size, not yet studied in detail (D. F. Anderson, unpublished). Hanson asked what cellular mechanism was involved; was this due to the increase in wall stress? Thornburg replied that in fetuses with increased right ventricular load, but without left ventricular hypertension or increased wall stress, the left ventricle grows faster, with large and more binucleate cells. Possible humoral factors should be considered. So the problem of ventricular growth is more complex and more interesting. He also mentioned that simple application of Laplace's law to the heart gave reasonable prediction of wall stress, even when used for instantaneous calculations of the gross changes during ejection.

John Challis and Evan Simpson asked whether attempts had been successful in growing myocytes in culture. Thornburg replied that culture in motionless conditions was unsatisfactory; the cells did not look like those in vivo. However, myocytes will attach to a plastic film, which when stretched rhythmically induces faster growth and histological changes which are more natural (Cooper et al., 1986).

References

Cooper G, Mercer HC, Hooper JK et al. (1986) Circ Res 58: 692–705.
Fisher DJ, Heymann MA, Rudolph AM (1982) Am J Physiol 242: H657–661.
Iwamato HS, Rudolph AM, Mirkin BL et al. (1983) Am J Physiol 245: H767–772.
Reed KL, Anderson CF, Shenker L (1987) Am J Obstet Gynecol 157: 774–779.
Reller MD, Morton MJ, Giraud GG et al. (1989) J Dev Physiol (in press).
Sahn DJ, Lange WL, Allen HD et al. (1980) Circ 62: 588–597.
Wladimiroff JW and McGhie J (1980) Br J Obstet Gynaec 88: 870–875.

4

The Intrauterine Origins of Adult Hypertension

D. J. P. BARKER

MRC Environmental Epidemiology Unit, Southampton General Hospital, Southampton, UK

There is increasing evidence that an adverse intrauterine environment has an important effect on the later risk of cardiovascular disease, i.e. ischaemic heart disease and stroke. Within England and Wales the large differences in rates of cardiovascular disease from place to place correlate strongly with differences in neonatal mortality 60 and more years ago (Barker and Osmond, 1986; Barker et al., 1989a). Most neonatal deaths at that time occurred during the first week after birth and were attributed to 'prematurity', i.e. low birthweight. This pointer to a relation with the intrauterine environment is reinforced by the geographical relation between cardiovascular disease and past maternal mortality, a relation which is especially strong for stroke (Barker and Osmond, 1987). Studies carried out in the early years of this century showed that in areas of Britain with high maternal mortality, mothers had poor physique, including shorter stature, and worse general health.

These ecological findings have been strongly supported by the results of a follow-up study of a group of men born around 1920 whose weights in infancy were recorded at the time (Barker et al., 1989c). The men were born in the county of Hertfordshire, England, where from 1911 onwards all babies, whether born at home or in hospital, were weighed at birth and followed up to one year of age. A total of 7991 men born in six districts during 1911–30 were identified: 5654 (71%) were traced, of whom 1186 died as adults. Death rates from ischaemic heart disease were highest in those with the lowest weight at one year. In Table 1 death rates are expressed in relation to a national average of 100 and standardized for age and sex. The overall standardized mortality ratio for Hertfordshire is 82. Ratios fall from 111 in men who weighed 18 pounds or less at one year, to 42 in those who weighed 27 pounds or more.

Fetal Autonomy and Adaptation. Edited by G. S. Dawes, A. Zacutti, F. Borruto and A. Zacutti, Jr
© 1990 John Wiley & Sons Ltd

TABLE 1 Standardized mortality ratios from ischaemic heart disease according to weight at one year in 5654 men

Weight (pounds)	Number of men	Mortality ratios
< 18	324	111
19–20	971	81
21–22	1850	98
23–24	1464	71
25–26	769	68
> 27	276	42
Total	5654	82

Both prenatal and postnatal growth were important in determining weight at one year, since few infants with below-average birthweights reached the heaviest weights at one. The combination of poor prenatal and postnatal growth led to the highest death rates: men who weighed 5.5 pounds or less at birth and 18 pounds or less at one year had a standardized mortality ratio of 220. Among the men who were exclusively bottle fed (7.6%) heavier weight at one was not associated with lower mortality. Figure 1 shows the relative risk of death from ischaemic heart disease among the breast-fed men according to birthweight and weight at one year.

Evidence that blood pressure is one of the links between the intrauterine environment and risk of cardiovascular disease comes from the inverse relation between birthweight and adult blood pressure (Barker et al., 1989b). Table 2 shows mean systolic blood pressures of 3259 men and women aged 36 years who were followed up from birth. These people are a national sample selected from all births occurring in Britain during one week in 1946. In Table 2 subjects are divided into three roughly equal groups by birthweight within each third of body weight. Among men, within each body weight group, mean systolic pressure fell by 2.6 mmHg from the lowest to the highest birthweight group. Among women the fall was 1.8 mmHg. There was no similar trend for diastolic pressure. In the national sample of 9921 10-year-old boys and girls there was a similar, though weaker, inverse relation between systolic blood pressure and birthweight.

I now report the preliminary results of a survey designed to examine more closely the relation between adult blood pressure and parameters of fetal growth. This survey was carried out with my colleagues Dr A. Bull and Dr C. Osmond (Barker et al., 1990). At a maternity hospital in Preston, a northern industrial town in England, detailed clinical records on every woman admitted to the delivery ward have been preserved for many years. Information was recorded in a standardized way and included measurements of the mother, of the infant at birth and

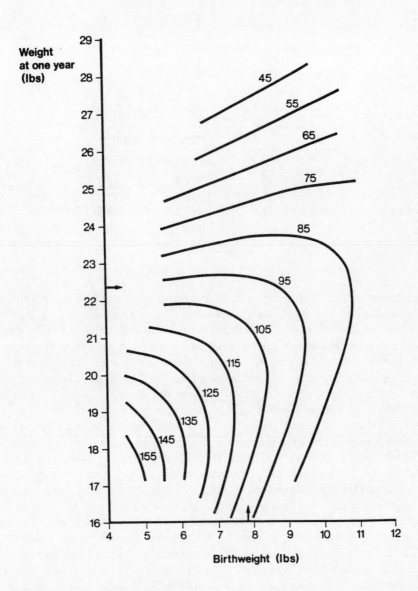

FIGURE 1   Relative risk for ischaemic heart disease in men who were breast fed according to birthweight and weight at one year. Lines join points with equal risk. Arrows = mean weight. From Barker et al., 1989c. Reproduced by permission of The Lancet Ltd.

TABLE 2   Mean systolic blood pressures (mmHg) of 1625 men and 1634 women at age 36 stratified by thirds of weight and birthweight

MEN	Current weight (kg)			
Birthweight	<71.1	71.1–80.0	>80.0	All men
Lowest	123.2	124.2	124.6	124.0
Middle	122.2	121.2	125.6	122.8
Highest	121.3	119.8	123.2	121.5
All	122.4	122.0	124.4	122.9
WOMEN	Current weight (kg)			
Birthweight	<56.6	56.6–64.5	>64.5	All women
Lowest	118.7	117.3	120.2	118.6
Middle	117.5	115.0	117.1	116.7
Highest	116.8	115.3	118.6	116.7
All	117.8	116.1	118.6	117.4

placental weight. Maternal measurements included external pelvimetry; infant measurements included weight, length, head circumference and biparietal and other head diameters. Identification data on the mother and child were sufficient to allow the children to be traced through the Central Register of the National Health Service. We have traced 259 children born from 1935 to 1938 who are still alive and live in or around Preston. The 139 men and 120 women were visited at home by a nurse who measured their height, weight, abdominal and hip girth, and blood pressure. Blood pressure was measured using a Dinamap automated recorder and was recorded twice, before and after an interview. At interview the person's medical history, current medication, smoking habits and alcohol consumption were recorded.

Table 3 shows the average of the two values of systolic blood pressure in relation to birthweight and placental weight. Consistent with previous observations the systolic pressure fell with increasing birthweight. However, this relation was small compared with the rise in pressure associated with increasing placental weight. Systolic pressure rose from 148 mmHg in those with the lightest placentas to 160.8 mmHg in those with the heaviest. This trend, which was statistically significant ($p < 0.001$), was seen within each birthweight group, and in both men and women. Mean systolic pressures in men rose from 146.7 mmHg in those with the lightest placentas to 159.2 mmHg in those with the heaviest. The corresponding values for women were 149.2 and 163.3. Diastolic pressures rose with placental weight but there was no trend with birthweight. The blood pressure values were little changed by adjustment for alcohol consumption and cigarette smoking.

TABLE 3 Systolic blood pressure (mmHg) in 259 men and women in relation to birthweight and placental weight

Birthweight (pounds)	Placental weight (ounces)				
	17 or less	18–20	21–24	25 +	All weights
≤5.5	150.2	146.4	155.4	207.0	152.3 (29)
5.5–6.4	148.0	152.9	152.9	177.6	153.8 (69)
6.5–7.5	148.2	151.7	145.1	163.0	150.8 (90)
≥7.5	140.2	151.0	149.2	155.3	151.5 (71)
All weights	148.0 (49)	151.6 (84)	149.1 (77)	160.8 (49)	151.9 (259)

Figures in brackets are numbers of people.

The strong relation between placental weight and adult blood pressure shown in this study needs confirmation. A further sample of men and women born in Preston is currently being examined. This second survey will be completed within two months. If it confirms the first survey we will need to examine the mechanisms whereby fetal blood pressure becomes elevated in association with (1) higher placental weight and (2) at each placental weight, lower birthweight.

References

Barker DJP and Osmond C (1986) Infant mortality, childhood nutrition, and ischaemic heart disease in England and Wales. Lancet i: 1077–1081.

Barker DJP and Osmond C (1987) Death rates from stroke in England and Wales predicted from past maternal mortality. Br Med J 295: 83–86.

Barker DJP, Osmond C, Law C (1989a) The intra-uterine and early postnatal origins of cardiovascular disease and chronic bronchitis. J Epidemiol Community Health 43: 237–240.

Barker DJP, Osmond C, Golding J, Kuh D, Wadsworth MEJ (1989b) Growth in utero, blood pressure in childhood and adult life, and mortality from cardiovascular disease. Br Med J 298: 564–567.

Barker DJP, Winter PD, Osmond C, Margetts B, Simmonds SJ (1989c) Weight in infancy and death from ischaemic heart disease. Lancet ii: 577–580.

Barker DJP, Bull AR, Osmond C, Simmonds SJ (1990) The effect of fetal and placental size on the risk of hypertension in adult life. Br Med J (in press).

Discussion

War Service and Smoking

Patrick wondered whether the results might have been distorted by the consequences of war service during 1914–18 or 1939–45, or by smoking. Barker explained that of his first group, born in Hertfordshire in the period 1910–30, some had died in childhood or as young adults and some had emigrated, but 75% of those sought were identified, an unusually high figure for long-term follow-up studies. The second group were born in Preston in 1935–8 and so the question of war service did not arise. Smoking in women was rare before World War II and so maternal smoking is unlikely to have been important. In the earlier Hertfordshire group the weight at one year did not predict lung cancer, suggesting that there was no relationship between infant growth and subsequent smoking. In the later Preston group smoking was only weakly related to blood pressure in the adults sampled. Drinking alcohol was more strongly related. But the strongest predictor of high blood pressure was placental weight.

Age at Birth

Mandruzzato asked whether there was a relation between ischaemic heart disease in adult life and either pre-term delivery or small size for gestational age at birth. Barker replied that for births in Hertfordshire there were no data on gestation. In Preston gestational age could only be deduced from the last menstrual period, information on which was only available in 75% of the cases. The numbers were as yet too small for the evidence to be secure, but there seemed to be an association between prolonged gestation and subsequent blood pressure. Additional data were required to clarify this point.

Genetic Factors

Redman asked whether the association between hypertension in adults and placental weight might be genetically determined. Barker did not think this likely. Hypertension in pregnant women did not give rise to greater placental weight, rather the contrary. The fact that hypertension is often familial does not necessarily mean that it must be genetically determined. There were other plausible possibilities. The stability of fetal growth rates through successive generations is thought to be due, at least in part, to an effect of the intrauterine environment on adult size and hence on growth in the next generation. Redman replied that pregnancy was associated with two types of hypertension, chronic hypertension preceding pregnancy and pre-eclampsia. Women with chronic hypertension were larger in height and weight, which would be associated with larger fetuses and placentas; placental weight and function appeared to be unaffected unless pre-eclampsia developed. However, he did not know specifically whether placental weight was *greater* in association with chronic maternal hypertension.

Bottle/Breast Feeding; Social Class

Ellendorff was surprised at the effects of bottle feeding. Barker confirmed that bottle-fed babies with high weight at one year did not have reduced ischaemic heart disease as adults; they were not protected. More evidence is needed on this point. A possible explanation was that such bottle-fed babies weighed more because they were fatter, as compared with breast-fed babies, who were longer.

Hanson suggested that social class was a strong predictor of ischaemic heart disease. He wondered whether the differences which Barker had described would disappear if the data were re-analysed for social class, for if so it might indicate that the processes he had discovered were fundamental, as opposed to a correlation. Barker replied that Hertfordshire *at the time in question* was a rural county in which social class was relatively unrelated to health. In the population studied social class at death was not related to infant weight. In the studies of survivors now under way the social class of those interviewed will be known, and can be related to infant weight, blood pressure, and other factors carrying a risk of ischaemic heart disease.

Placental Size

Visser remarked that Barker's data showed that large placental weight had a stronger effect in predicting hypertension than did low birthweight in predicting ischaemic heart disease. He deduced that malnutrition in utero could not be an important factor, and wondered whether the combination of a large placenta with lower birthweight might be a consequence of a disorder in early development. Pardi asked how many of these smaller babies with large placentas had cardiac problems. Barker replied that as adults they did not have cardiovascular anomalies except that some had ischaemic heart disease; they were otherwise normal, though at birth they had short length in relation to head circumference. To him they seemed to be infants with larger growth aspirations than were attainable. In reply to a question from Ellendorff on maternal parity, Barker said that this was not available in the data from Hertfordshire. It was an interesting point that was being examined in the Preston data.

Barker agreed with Patrick's comment that he had made an implicit assumption as to the connection between hypertension and ischaemic heart disease; there was, however, strong evidence for this association. Patrick asked whether there were data on the mechanisms which determine fetal vascular growth (in the myocardium and elsewhere) in response to environmental changes. With Thornburg he speculated that the peripheral vasculature, its collagen and elastin for example, might be developed in late fetal life to fit the current arterial pressure, determined in part by the relative sizes of the placenta and fetus. Though there was much evidence, in animals and man, to show a close relationship between fetal and placental weight, the principles which determined divergence from this close relationship in late fetal life, after the placenta had reached its greatest weight, had not been investigated. The facts reported suggested that this was worth new study.

* * *

Discussion on Barker's paper was resumed after Dr Redman had presented his paper on the origin of the placenta and Dr Cetin had referred to the possibility that the placenta could steal amino acids from the fetus with growth retardation.

Adult Blood Pressure and Placental Weight

Thornburg thought it far fetched that a short-term adaptation of a fetus in trouble would have such a long-term effect on the likelihood of ischaemic heart disease in adult life. Barker rehearsed the main points in favour of his hypothesis. The inverse relation between birthweight and arterial pressure had been established in:

1. A national sample of 3200 adult men and women in Britain.
2. 9900 10-year-old children.
3. 7000 5-to-6-year-old children.
4. Two smaller samples of younger children.

Whatever the causal connection, this relationship was now well-established. His data on the placenta were more limited (but would be doubled within two months). There was already evidence of a much higher systolic pressure *when the placenta was large*. At any placental weight the arterial blood pressure was less with greater fetal weight and length at birth.

Dawes remarked that Barker was describing a particular subset of small babies, not tiny but toward the lower end of the frequency distribution at term, recognizable at birth by their relatively large placenta and low length : head circumference ratio. Barker added that they were also recognizable in later life by being short, fatter, and with a higher blood pressure. In an obstetric database they might well be invisible.

Redman and Mandruzzato pointed out the problems with placental weight measurements, which were crude because of inconsistencies in the way in which the placenta was handled and trimmed, still perhaps retaining maternal or fetal blood. The data were crude but could be examined. Even if imprecise they might still be useful. Pardi wondered whether the data were disturbed by infection, especially on delivery at 36–37 weeks gestation. And Visser was still concerned about the effects of smoking. Nevertheless, Barker stuck to his hypothesis, which of course must be validated by further measurements. Even if the placenta is not weighed with the loving care of the baby (Dawes wondered how often the scales were calibrated) his preliminary figures had shown an unexpected relationship with placental weight, which raised new and unexpected causal possibilities.

The Control of Placental Growth

Dawes wondered what was known of the control of placental growth. This seemed to be a neglected subject. Many meetings and reviews had been concerned with the determinants of fetal growth, but few had thought it worthwhile considering the problem of placental growth. It was only recently that hormones other than progesterone had been recognized in the placenta, and that convincing evidence had accumulated as to placental involvement in the initiation of labour. The placenta reached its maximum weight early in gestation in many species, though further morphological changes continued thereafter. On average there was a close relation between placental and fetal weight, which suggested appropriate adjustment, perhaps on either side. Challis referred to the compensatory growth of the primary placenta of the rhesus monkey (Hill, 1974), which occurred when the umbilical vessels to the secondary (smaller) placenta were tied, suggesting an active process. Dawes also referred to the work of Alexander (1964), who produced growth retardation in fetal sheep by cauterizing 80% of the uterine caruncles to which the placentomes are attached. The few placentomes which do develop in these circumstances also show signs of adjustment, by eversion of the placentomal cups. Many of the placentomes become unusually large. It was uncertain how this was effected, by local growth hormones or otherwise; the stimulus was not known. The problem usually proposed was one of fetal adaptation to placental size; the converse had not been considered but it was a good biological problem.

Patrick returned to the clinical problem. Access to an obstetric database might be helpful, but formulation of the questions which should be asked was not so simple as it at first appeared.

References

Alexander G (1964) J Reprod Fertil 7: 307–322.
Hill DE (1974) In: Size at Birth. Ciba Foundation Symposium 27, pp 99–125.

5

Adaptation to Vibroacoustic Stimulation

J. PATRICK* AND R. GAGNON
Departments of Obstetrics/Gynaecology and of Physiology,
University of Western Ontario, Lawson Research Institute

During the past five years, considerable interest has developed in the use of of external sound and vibration to measure responses in human fetuses as a method of assessing fetal health. The purpose of this chapter will be to review, during gestation, fetal auditory and vibratory sensory development and responses. An underlying objective will be to emphasize the paucity of information on the fetal mechanisms involved in the response to vibroacoustic stimulation. Further, concerns regarding safety of the test in practice and the clinical evidence of usefulness of the response will be addressed.

Development of Fetal Vibroacoustic Receptors

The primitive embryonic ear forms from an ectodermal thickening known as the auditory placode (Altmann, 1950). The otocyst is formed by invagination of the auditory placode into surrounding mesenchyme. In the 4–5 week human embryo the otocyst divides into two lobes. One lobe becomes the cochlea and the other the labyrinth (Ormerod, 1960). By 6 months of fetal age, both the organ of Corti and the tunnel of Corti are present in the turns of the cochlea. Studies in premature human neonates have suggested that pathways exist to process auditory sensory information by about 30 weeks gestation (Sammons, 1980).

Meissner's and Pacinian corpuscles are peripheral vibration-sensitive endings which transmit vibrotactile stimuli. It has been reported that these sensory receptors are present in the hands of human fetuses by 24 weeks gestation.

---

*Deceased

Fetal Autonomy and Adaptation. Edited by G. S. Dawes, A. Zacutti, F. Borruto and A. Zacutti, Jr
©1990 John Wiley & Sons Ltd

The adult ear responds to sound frequencies in the range of 20–20,000 Hz. Schmidt (1986) reported the optimal response occurs around 2000 Hz. The ear is designed to receive sounds transmitted in air and can be considered an impedance-matching organ. The function of the ear depends on the external auditory canal, the tympanic membrane, and the bony ossicles that link the membrane to the fluid canals of the inner ear.

During fetal life, the middle ear and external auditory canal are filled with fluid. This should tend to dampen the frequency response of the tympanic membrane and ossicles and may diminish the ability of the middle ear to perform impedance-matching. Based on this logic, it has been supposed that fetuses might require high sound pressure levels in order to detect sound.

One method of documenting hearing function is the measurement of auditory brain responses (ABRs), which are neuroelectrical waves recorded from EEG electrodes placed on the scalp of newborns (Despland and Galambos, 1980). ABRs have been measured between 26 and 28 weeks gestation in human newborns but have not been detected before 26 weeks. During elegant experiments conducted in chronic fetal lamb preparations, Woods et al. (1984) have demonstrated maturational changes in the development of ABRs during the last third of pregnancy.

The data from lamb experiments and from human newborns would suggest that an adequate sound stimulus that exceeds background noise in utero could be detected and, therefore, elicit fetal responses by 26 weeks gestational age.

The Fetal Sound Environment

During pregnancy in sheep, Vince et al. (1980, 1985), using a miniaturized radio hydrophone implanted on the fetal neck, measured intrauterine background noise of 60 dB with a maximum attenuation of sound across the uterine and abdominal walls of 25 dB at a frequency of 5000 Hz. Intrauterine background noise apparently originates from the maternal gastrointestinal system but not the cardiovascular system. In addition, maternal vocalization results in periodic increases in background noise.

During human pregnancy, Walker et al. (1971) reported intrauterine background sound pressure levels of 82 dB, which seemed to be related to blood flow and muscle movement. Their measurements were made with a microphone placed beside the fetal head in pregnant women during labour. Recent reports by Querleu et al. (1986), using different recording methods, reported intra-amniotic sound pressure levels of 28–95 dB. It is important that Walker et al. measured an attenuation of sound by the maternal abdominal and uterine tissues of at least 40 dB at frequencies > 1000 Hz. Both Walker and Querleu made use of intrauterine microphones placed in different locations with different size and frequency response characteristics. Recordings made from intrauterine microphones covered with rubber made during human labour by Querleu have clearly demonstrated that mother's voice and the normal speaking voice of investigators present in the room can be detected in utero. These observations suggest that attenuation of sound across the maternal abdominal and uterine tissues may be much less than was previously supposed.

Transmission of Vibroacoustic Stimulation to the Fetus

In North America, vibroacoustic stimulation of human fetuses is widely used for assessing fetal health. The instrument is placed on the surface of the maternal abdomen over the fetal head in order to elicit fetal responses. The electronic artificial larynx (Western Electric, Model 5C, New York) produces a broad-band noise with multiple harmonics up to 10,000 Hz (Gagnon et al., 1986). A maximum sound pressure level, measured in air at 1 cm from the surface of the instrument, is 110 dB at 10,000 Hz. The surface of the instrument vibrates at frequencies between 10 and 20,000 Hz, with a maximum vibration pressure occurring at 450 Hz.

Initially, investigators considered this to be a reasonable stimulus for use during human pregnancy, based on the attenuation data of Walker et al. (1971). However, the characteristics of sound and vibration may actually be amplified using this device. Gerhardt et al. (1988) placed a hydrophone inside the uterine cavity of pregnant sheep and reported a sound pressure level of 135 dB during stimulation on the surface of the maternal abdomen with an electronic artificial larynx. These investigators recommended caution in administering a vibroacoustic stimulus during human pregnancy until the effects of high sound pressure levels on the fetus are better understood. It will be important to make similar measurements during human pregnancy and to determine whether actual harm could result from exposure of fetuses to intense sound stimulation at different gestational ages.

Fetal 'Behaviour'

Developments in the technology of ultrasound over the past 15 years have permitted measurement, during human pregnancy, of fetal breathing, eye and body movements, fetal heart rate and heart rate variability, and of blood flow velocimetry during human pregnancy. Assessment of the fetal adaptation to sound and vibration has been based on observations of changes in these measurements following vibroacoustic stimulation of the human fetus in utero. Before considering the changes produced by vibroacoustic stimulation on human behaviour, it is important to review the physiology, which has been derived from controlled experiments in fetal animals and human observational studies.

Fetal Electrocortical Function

Dawes et al. (1972) first reported measurement of the fetal electrocorticogram (ECOG) after 125 days gestation (term, 147 days) in sheep. They recognized two characteristic patterns of ECOG. Episodes of a high-voltage, low-frequency ECOG alternated with episodes of low-voltage, high-frequency wave patterns. Based on direct observations of animals delivered into saline baths, the high-voltage pattern appeared to represent a time of fetal quiet sleep and the low-voltage pattern was recorded both during times of fetal sleep characterized by eye movements and during times of fetal wakefulness. Numerous reports have demonstrated that, during late gestation in sheep, animals spend about 50% of the time in a low-voltage pattern and about 50% of the time in a high-voltage pattern. Ruckebusch (1972) reported the presence of fetal wakefulness in mature fetal lambs about 6% of the time.

It is important that fetal biophysical measurements are clustered according to the presence or absence of one or other electrocortical pattern. In sheep, episodic fetal breathing movements and rapid eye movements occur only during low-voltage ECOG (Dawes et al., 1972). During these times, fetal heart rate and heart rate variability are usually increased (Dalton et al., 1977). In sheep, Natale et al. (1981) reported that fetal forelimb movements often increase during times of change from one electrocortical pattern to another. Richardson et al. (1985) measured a 28% increase in cerebral cortical oxidative metabolism during low-voltage electrocortical activity compared to high-voltage activity. They also reported dramatic increases in blood flow to the pons, medulla and brainstem during low-voltage electrocortical patterns.

Therefore, evidence from fetal lamb experiments demonstrates that in the mature fetal lamb, measurements of fetal breathing movements, eye movements, body movements, heart rate and brain blood flow are modulated by episodes of fetal electrocortical activity. During human pregnancy it has not yet been feasible to make direct measurements of fetal electrocortical activity. It has been suggested (Nijhuis et al., 1982) that the clustering of state dependent variables, such as fetal eye movements, body movements, and heart rate variability, might reflect the presence of normal fetal cortical function.

Human Fetal 'Behavioural States'

Evidence that similar periodicities in electrocortical activity exist during human pregnancy has come from several sources. Rosen et al. (1973) recorded the EEG from human fetuses during labour and reported similar waveform patterns of quiet sleep, active sleep and awake state to those measured in newborns. Further, the classic work of Prechtl (1975) demonstrated that clustering of variables such as body movements, heart rate variability, and eye movements could define five separate states of activity during newborn life. Using Prechtl's criteria in the newborn, Nijhuis et al. (1982) measured episodes of rapid eye movements in human fetuses during the last eight weeks of pregnancy and classified fetal activity patterns into four fetal 'behavioural states'.

An underlying assumption in the measurement of fetal behavioural states is that these states may reflect fetal cortical function. It is assumed that fetal cortical function might be an important marker of fetal hypoxia and therefore useful in the assessment of fetal health. Unfortunately, recent studies have demonstrated that this assumption may not be valid. Cohn et al. (1974) first reported that the mature fetal lamb was able to maintain oxygen delivery to brain tissue by redistributing blood flow towards the brain at the expense of flow to non-essential organs such as skeletal muscle and body mass. Their observations were made during late fetal life in sheep over short observation intervals. We recently extended the observations of Cohn et al. by developing a method for prolonged administration of hypoxia to pregnant ewes and have demonstrated that the fetus is able to maintain cerebral oxidative metabolism during hypoxia with increasing metabolic acidosis. Indeed, our measurements indicate that fetal cerebral oxidative metabolism is unchanged down to arterial pH levels of 7.15 and that fetal electrocortical activity continues a normal pattern of cycling (Richardson et al., 1989). Therefore, normal fetal cortical function may be a very poor sign of fetal hypoxia.

A further problem in the use of fetal behavioural parameters to indicate fetal cortical function is that despite the fact that these parameters are clustered according to electrocortical state they also have separate mechanisms of control, which may alter the incidence or occurrence within selected electrocortical states.

Fetal Breathing Movements

Dawes et al. (1972) measured fetal breathing movements in sheep and recognized that breathing movements were episodic and occurred only during times of low-voltage electrocortical activity. Fetal breathing movements are increased in incidence during fetal hypercapnia and decreased during fetal hypoxia (Boddy et al., 1974; Adamson et al., 1985). These changes are independent of changes in fetal electrocortical activity. Similarly, fetal breathing movements are stimulated by inhibitors of prostaglandin synthesis (Kitterman et al., 1979) and the incidence of breathing movements is reduced prior to the onset of spontaneous labour. These changes are also independent of any change in electrocortical activity.

Fetal Body Movements

During late pregnancy in sheep fetal forelimb movements were measured by Natale et al. (1981), who reported that experimentally induced hypoxaemia virtually abolished all activity. Under the conditions of this experiment it would be assumed from other data that fetal electrocortical activity was unchanged and that fetal cerebral oxidative metabolism was maintained. These studies further demonstrate the dissociation of controls of fetal body movements from underlying patterns of electrocortical function.

Fetal Eye Movements

Under the conditions of our experiments (Richardson et al., 1989) fetal hypoxia resulted in arrest of fetal electro-ocular activity. This occurred during times of normal fetal electrocortical function as indicated by electrical measurements and by fetal cerebral oxidative metabolism.

Behavioural state studies during human pregnancy rely on the measurement of fetal eye movements. It is known that rapid eye movements occur only during low-voltage electrocortical activity in mature fetal lamb experiments, and that rapid eye movements are closely correlated with rapid-eye-movement sleep in studies of human newborns. As has been demonstrated above, fetal rapid eye movements can be dissociated from fetal electrocortical function under the conditions of hypoxia. Furthermore, studies from our laboratory (Patrick et al., 1985) have demonstrated the suppression of rapid eye movements during late pregnancy in sheep by maternal ethanol infusion. Rapid eye movements did not correlate with fetal electrocortical activity under the conditions of these experiments. Finally, it is important to note that recent data have demonstrated that certain hypoxic conditions resulting in diminished fetal breathing activity or fetal rapid eye movement activity have different time courses of effect on these measurements. For example, Bocking et al. (1988) induced fetal hypoxaemia by reducing maternal uterine arterial blood flow over a period of 48 hours in sheep. Under the conditions of their experiment, fetal rapid eye movement activity returned hours before the return of fetal breathing movements. If this fact is confirmed during human pregnancy, it would further confuse the use of clustering of biophysical variables as a marker of fetal behavioural state.

Summary

Information obtained from carefully controlled experiments in late pregnancy in sheep suggest that under normal conditions the clustering of variables such as rapid eye movements, fetal breathing activity, body movements and heart rate changes can be used as a reasonable indicator of fetal electrocortical function. However, under conditions of hypoxia and of numerous other physiological stimuli, biophysical variables are dissociated from electrocortical activity and from each other in time. It is against this background that human observational studies of effects of vibroacoustic stimulation must be considered.

Effects of Vibroacoustic Stimulation on Fetal Measurements

Fetal Heart Rate

It has been known since 1964 (Johansson et al., 1964), that fetal heart rate (FHR) increases in response to loud sound stimulation from transducers placed on the surface of the maternal abdomen. Since that time there have been numerous reports of FHR response to sound of different frequencies, durations and pressure levels (Dwornicka et al., 1964; Grimwade et al., 1971; Read et al., 1977; Luz et al., 1980; Davey et al., 1984; Jensen, 1984; Querleu et al., 1984).

Based on these reports, we conducted a series of carefully controlled experiments in 83 healthy pregnant women volunteers between 26 and 40 weeks gestational age. FHR analysis was conducted using a Hewlett Packard 8040A monitor and on-line computerized analysis, using the method of Dawes et al. (1985). Studies were conducted in a quiet room with women in a left lateral recumbent position or sitting up. Subjects were given an 800 Kcal meal and after one hour studies were commenced. A one-hour control period was followed by application of the electronic artificial larynx (EAL) over the fetal head with a 5-second vibroacoustic stimulus. Control groups received a similar stimulus on the maternal hand.

The FHR response to vibroacoustic stimulation was dependent on gestational age. After 30 weeks gestation there was a prolonged and significant increase in the mean FHR. Near term, the increase in FHR was prolonged for up to 1 hour. It is important that neither maternal heart rate nor blood pressure were influenced by the stimulation. Between 26 and 30 weeks, the FHR response to stimulation consisted of a single prolonged FHR acceleration. In this age group there was no increase in the number of fetal heart rate accelerations following stimulation. Conversely, in fetuses more than 33 weeks gestation there was an increase in the number of FHR accelerations between 10 and 20 minutes following stimulus (Gagnon et al., 1987a, 1988d). It is important that the increase in the number of FHR accelerations did not occur until 10 minutes following stimuli. Therefore, the effects of vibroacoustic stimulation on the fetal heart rate are dependent on gestational age in human fetuses.

Fetal Body Movements

It was originally reported by Gelman et al. (1982) that an increase in fetal movements occurs following a vibroacoustic stimulus applied on the surface of the maternal abdomen over a period of 1 minute. Later, Schmidt et al. (1985) reported no changes in fetal activity or heart rate when a loud sound stimulus was applied without touching the maternal abdomen.

We pursued these observations by measuring fetal breathing and body movements before or after a 5-second vibroacoustic stimulation with the EAL under conditions mentioned above in healthy selected women volunteers between 26 and 40 weeks gestational age (Gagnon et al., 1987b, 1988a). In fetuses between 33 and 40 weeks gestational age there was an increase in gross fetal body movements which began 10 minutes following the stimulus and persisted for up to 1 hour (Gagnon et al., 1987b). However, in fetuses between 26 and 32 weeks gestation (Gagnon et al., 1988a) gross fetal body movements were not altered by the stimulus.

Fetal Breathing Movements

Under the conditions of our experiments, fetal breathing activity was altered only in fetuses between 36 and 40 weeks gestational age (Gagnon et al., 1987b). Following stimulation with the EAL, the incidence of fetal breathing movements immediately decreased and examination of histograms of breath-breath intervals indicated breathing activity became more irregular for a period of up to 1 hour following a 5-second vibroacoustic stimulus. Fetal breathing movements were not influenced in fetuses of 26–35 weeks gestational age.

Vibroacoustic Stimulation in Growth-Restricted Fetuses

Growth-Restricted Fetuses of 32–40 Weeks Gestational Age

In order to determine responses to vibroacoustic stimulation in growth-restricted human fetuses we recruited a group of 17 pregnant women of 34–40 weeks gestational age that subsequently delivered a baby of birthweight less than the third percentile (Gagnon et al., 1988b). Twenty-five healthy pregnant women with normally grown infants matched for gestational age were used as controls. The umbilical cord arterial blood gas values demonstrated that the 17 growth-restricted fetuses were not acidaemic at birth but had a slightly lower PO2 (less by a mean value of 3 mmHg) than the normally grown controls. Studies were conducted as mentioned above.

Prior to vibroacoustic stimulation the growth-restricted fetuses demonstrated a 40% decrease in the incidence of gross fetal body movements and a 25% decrease in long-term FHR variability. However, fetal heart rate and fetal activity patterns following stimulation with EAL in the growth-restricted fetuses were not different from those in the normally grown fetuses. These data suggest that fetal responses to EAL could not be used to differentiate the late-onset severely growth-restricted human fetus from normally grown fetuses.

Intrauterine Growth Restriction Before 32 Weeks Gestational Age

In order to determine the effects of EAL on human fetuses with severe early-onset intrauterine growth restriction, we recruited nine pregnant volunteers for study prior to 32 weeks gestation, who delivered infants on average at 32.8 weeks gestation that were less than the third centile for birthweight in our population (Gagnon et al., 1989). All infants survived the neonatal period and none exhibited congenital anomalies. Eight of the nine infants had a normal umbilical arterial pH and one was delivered with an arterial pH of 7.04. Infants were matched with a control group of normally grown fetuses at the same gestational age.

Before stimulation the nine fetuses exhibited diminished fetal heart rate variability, fetal heart rate accelerations and fetal movements. We did not demonstrate any significant effect of vibroacoustic stimulation on either the mean fetal heart rate or fetal movement patterns in the nine fetuses with early-onset growth restriction. The data suggested that, in this small group, a delay in maturation of fetal sensory receptors or brainstem function might have occurred.

Umbilical Arterial Blood Flow Velocity

In order to determine the effects of vibroacoustic stimulation on umbilical arterial blood flow velocity waveform patterns we (Gagnon et al., 1988c) studied 12 healthy pregnant volunteers of 37–41 weeks gestational age. Following a 5-second vibroacoustic stimulation with the EAL, there was a significant decrease in the S/D ratio of the umbilical arterial waveform for a period of 5 minutes after stimulus. Analysis of the mean fetal heart rate during Doppler measurements indicated the decrease in umbilical arterial S/D waveform ratio was related to fetal tachycardia and not to changes in placental vascular resistance.

Effects of Vibration on the Human Fetus

Concerns regarding possible adverse effects of loud noise on human fetal development have recently led us to study the effects of low-frequency vibration (100 Hz, square wave) as a stimulus applied on the surface of the maternal abdomen during late human gestation. Preliminary data suggest that application of low-frequency vibration can induce a switch in fetal behaviour from a quiet state, during which no gross fetal body movements or fetal eye movements are observed, to an active state during which fetal eye movements and body movements and heart rate accelerations are present. This response agrees with data reported by Hutt et al. (1969) in studies of newborn human infants. It remains to be determined if this less noxious stimulus might be clinically useful in assessment of fetal health.

Future Directions in the Study of Vibroacoustic Stimulation

It is perhaps unfortunate that vibroacoustic stimulation is already widely used in North America in the assessment of human fetal health. This chapter has demonstrated potential concerns regarding safety to the human fetus of exposure to loud intrauterine noise. It will be important to document intrauterine sound pressure levels during human pregnancy. The data of Gerhardt et al. (1988) from studies of sheep demonstrate extremely high intrauterine sound pressure levels during stimulation with the EAL. Further, no data have yet been published which examine the long-term auditory function of fetuses that have been exposed to sound stimulation in utero.

Published data demonstrate that dramatic effects on the fetal heart rate, fetal body movements, and fetal breathing movements result from stimulation with the EAL. No data are yet available to determine the mechanism of these effects. Therefore, there is a real need for development of a suitable animal model for understanding such mechanisms.

Finally, there are numerous reports in the recent literature regarding clinical use of the EAL in detection of fetal health. Unfortunately, no controlled clinical trials have yet been published which suggest any clinical benefit, as measured by improved perinatal outcome, from the use of EAL in clinical practice. It is prudent to conclude that the routine use of vibroacoustic stimulation in obstetrical care should be withheld until clear evidence of safety and benefit are established.

Acknowledgements

This work was supported by the Physicians' Services Incorporated Foundation, Ontario Ministry of Health, Medical Research Council of Canada, The Variety Club of Ontario. J. P. is a member of the Canadian Medical Research Council Group in Fetal and Neonatal Health and Development.

References

Adamson SL, Patrick JE, Challis JRG (1985) Effects of Naloxone on breathing, electrocortical, heart rate, glucose and cortical responses to hypoxia in the sheep fetus. J Devel Physiol 151: 283–287.

Altmann E (1950) Normal development of the ear and its mechanics. Arch Otolaryngol 52: 725.

Bocking AD, Gagnon R, Milne KM, White SE (1988) Behavioural activity during prolonged hypoxemia in fetal sheep. J Appl Physiol 65: 2420–2426.

Boddy K, Dawes GS, Fisher R, Printer S, Robinson JS (1974) Fetal respiratory movements, electrocortical and cardiovascular responses to hypoxaemia and hypercapnia in sheep. J Physiol 243: 599–618.

Cohn HE, Sacks EJ, Heymann MA et al. (1974) Cardiovascular responses to hypoxemia and acidemia in fetal lambs. Am J Obstet Gynecol 120: 817–824.

Dalton KJ, Dawes GS, Patrick JE (1977) Diurnal, respiratory and other rhythms of fetal heart rate in lambs. Am J Obstet Gynecol 127: 414–424.

Davey DA, Dommisse J, Macnab M et al. (1984) The value of an auditory stimulatory test in antenatal fetal cardiotocograph. Europ J Obstet Gynecol Reprod Biol 18: 273.

Dawes GS, Fox HE, Leduc BM et al. (1972) Respiratory movements and rapid eye movement sleep in the foetal lamb. J Physiol (Lond) 220: 119–143.

Dawes GS, Redman CWG, Smith JH (1985) Improvements in the registration and analysis of fetal heart rate records at the bedside. Br J Obstet Gynaecol 92: 317–325.

Despland PA and Galambos R (1980) The auditory brain stem response: A useful diagnostic tool in the intensive care nursery. Pediatr Res 14: 154.

Dwornicka B, Jasienska A, Smolarz W et al. (1964) Attempt of determining the fetal reaction to acoustic stimulation. Acta Otolaryngol 57: 571.

Gagnon R, Patrick J, Foreman J, West R (1986) Stimulation of human fetuses with sound and vibration. Am J Obstet Gynecol 155: 848.

Gagnon R, Hunse C, Carmichael L et al. (1987a) External vibratory acoustic stimulation near term: fetal heart rate and heart rate variability responses. Am J Obstet Gynecol 156: 323–327.

Gagnon R, Hunse C, Carmichael L et al. (1987b) Human fetal responses to vibratory acoustic stimulation from twenty-six weeks to term. Am J Obstet Gynecol 157: 1375–1381.

Gagnon R, Hunse C, Carmichael L et al. (1988a) Fetal heart rate and fetal activity patterns after vibratory acoustic stimulation at thirty to thirty-two weeks' gestational age. Am J Obstet Gynecol 158: 75–79.

Gagnon R, Hunse C, Fellows F et al. (1988b) Fetal heart rate and activity patterns in growth-retarded fetuses: Changes after vibratory acoustic stimulation. Am J Obstet Gynecol 158: 265–271.

Gagnon R, Morrow R, Ritchie K, Hunse C, Patrick J (1988c) Umbilical and uterine arterial blood flow velocities following vibratory acoustic stimulation. Am J Obstet Gynecol 159: 574–578.

Gagnon R, Hunse C, Patrick J (1988d) Fetal responses to vibratory acoustic stimulation: Influence of basal heart rate. Am J Obstet Gynecol 159: 835–839.

Gagnon R, Hunse C, Carmichael L, Patrick J (1989) Vibratory acoustic stimulation in 26- to 32-week, small-for-gestational-age fetus. Am J Obstet Gynecol 160: 160.

Gelman SR, Wood S, Spellacy WN et al. (1982) Fetal movements in response to sound stimulation. Am J Obstet Gynecol 143: 484–485.

Gerhardt KJ, Abrams RM, Kovaz BM et al. (1988) Intrauterine noise levels produced in pregnant ewes by sound applied to the abdomen. Am J Obstet Gynecol 159: 228.

Grimwade JG, Walker DW, Bartlett M et al. (1971) Human fetal heart rate change and movement in response to sound and vibration. Am J Obstet Gynecol 109: 86.

Hutt SJ, Lenard HG, Prechtl HFR (1969) Psychophysiological studies in newborn infants. Adv in Child Dev 4: 127–150.

Jensen OH (1984) Fetal heart rate response to controlled sound stimuli during the third trimester of normal pregnancy. Acta Obstet Gynecol Scand 63: 193.

Johansson B, Wedenberg E, Westin B (1964) Measurement of tone response by the human fetus. A preliminary report. Acta Otolaryngol 57: 188.

Kitterman JA, Liggins GC, Clements JA et al. (1979) Stimulation of breathing movements in fetal sheep by inhibitors of prostaglandin synthesis. J Develop Physiol 1: 453–466.

Luz NP, Lima CP, Luz SH et al. (1980) Auditory evoked responses of the human fetus. I. Behaviour during progress of labor. Acta Obstet Gynecol Scand 59: 395.

Natale R, Clelow F, Dawes GS (1981) Measurement of fetal forelimb movements in lambs in utero. Am J Obstet Gynecol 140: 545–551.

Nijhuis JG, Prechtl HFR, Martin CB, Bots RSGM (1982) Are there behavioural states in the human fetus? Early Hum Dev 6: 177.

Ormerod FC (1960) The pathology of congenital deafness in the child. In: The Modern Educational Treatment of Deafness (Ed: Ewing A), p 811. Manchester University Press, Manchester.

Patrick J, Richardson B, Hasen G et al. (1985) Effects of maternal ethanol infusion on fetal cardiovascular and brain activity in lambs. Am J Obstet Gynecol 151: 859.

Prechtl HFR (1975) Problems of behavioural studies in the newborn infant. In: Advances in the Study of Behaviour (Eds: Lehrman DS, Hinde RA, Shae E), Vol I. Academic Press, New York.

Querleu D, Boutteville C, Renard X (1984) Evaluation diagnostique de la souffrance foetale pendant la grossesse au moyen d'un test de stimulation sonore. J Gynecol Obstet Biol Reprod 13: 789.

Querleu D, Renard X, Versyp F (1986) Vie sensorielle du foetus. In: L'environnement de la Naissance (Eds: Tournaire M and Levy G), pp 15–41. Vigot, Paris.

Read JA and Miller FC (1977) Fetal heart rate acceleration in response to acoustic stimulation as a measure of fetal wellbeing. Am J Obstet Gynecol 129: 512.

Richardson BS, Patrick JE, Abduljabbar H (1985) Cerebral oxidative metabolism in the fetal lamb. Relationship to electrocortical state. Am J Obstet Gynecol 153: 426–431.

Richardson BS, Rurak D, Patrick JE et al. (1989) Cerebral oxidative metabolism during sustained hypoxemia in fetal sheep. J Develop Physiol 11: 37–43.

Rosen MG, Scibetta JJ, Chik L, Borgstedt AD (1973) An approach to the study of brain damage: the principles of fetal FEEG. Am J Obstet Gynecol 115: 37.

Ruckebusch Y (1972) Development of sleep and wakefulness in the foetal lamb. Electroencephalogr Clin Neurophysiol 32: 119–128.

Sammons WAH (1980) Premature behaviour and the neonatal intensive care unit environment. In: Manual of Neonatal Care (Eds: Cloherty JP and Stark AR), pp 359–363. Little Brown, Boston.

Schmidt RF (1986) Fundamentals of Sensory Physiology, 3rd edn. Springer Verlag, Berlin.

Schmidt W, Boos R, Gnirs J et al. (1985) Fetal behavioral states and controlled sound stimulation. Early Hum Devel 12: 145–153.

Vince MA and Armitage SE (1980) Sound stimulation available to the sheep foetus. Reprod Nutr Dev 20: 801.

Vince MA, Billing AE, Baldwin BA et al. (1985) Maternal vocalizations and other sounds in the fetal lamb's sound environment. Early Hum Devel 11: 179.

Walker DW, Grimwade JC, Wood C (1971) Intrauterine noise: a component of the fetal environment. Am J Obstet Gynecol 109: 91.

Woods JR, Plessinger M, Mack C (1984) The fetal auditory brainstem response. Pediatr Res 18: 83.

Discussion

Maternal Changes

In reply to a question from Ellendorff, Patrick said that vibroacoustic stimuli had no effect on *maternal* blood pressure or heart rate. He had not measured maternal plasma catecholamines or cortisol. Like many clinicians he supposed that maternal 'stress' might have an effect upon the fetus, by humoral effects across the placenta or through a change in uterine blood supply, but of this he had no proof. Visser then quoted an association of maternal excitement with an increase in fetal body movements over a 2-hour period of observation made by a Belgian psychologist (Van den Bergh et al., 1989). After a volcanic explosion in Italy, pregnant women had rushed to hospital with vigorous and continuous fetal movements; this was followed by absence of movements for 6–8 hours. Though anecdotal this evidence was suggestive.

Habituation and Sleep States

Ellendorff asked whether there were long-term effects of vibroacoustic stimuli. Patrick quoted the evidence of Leader who had studied 'habituation' in human fetuses over the past 10 years in South Africa, and more recently in sheep in Australia under the guidance of Professor E. Lumbers (Leader et al., 1988). There was a great variation in the number of brief stimuli, applied every 2 minutes, before habituation, defined as failure to respond, variation so great that its significance was doubtful. In the data so far published no account had been taken of sleep state in human fetuses, or of electrocorticographic activity in fetal sheep.

Redman asked whether Patrick had found a difference in response with sleep state in human fetuses using vibroacoustic stimuli. Patrick replied that the human response had three components. First there was always a 'startle', a brief fetal movement accompanied by a brief change in FHR rate, present from 24 weeks gestational age. From 28 weeks onwards there was also an immediate eye movement. Secondly there was a consistent change in sleep state (i.e. to state 2F if presently in state 1F), though the consequential increase in fetal movements was delayed by 10 minutes. Thirdly there was a large rise in FHR, and in FHR variation, of slow onset but continuing for up to an hour near term, attributed to humoral factors, possibly to catecholamine release.

If vibroacoustic stimuli were applied randomly they would occur more often in state 2F since this was present for 70% of the time near term. If applied during a cardiac acceleration (e.g. associated with a fetal movement) the heart rate increased yet further. He did not regard the large increase in heart rate (to a maximum value of 160 bpm) as cause for concern in normal fetuses, but was worried about the possible effects in severely growth-retarded fetuses if accompanied by a rise in plasma catecholamines.

Visser wondered whether the site of action of vibroacoustic stimuli was cochlear, vestibular or on proprioceptors. He favoured the latter two possibilities (however, see later discussion on animal studies, ed.) as a newborn infant in quiet sleep (state 1) does not respond to sound, but does so in rapid-eye-movement sleep (state 2). However, an alternative explanation might be a reaction to pain, as a newborn infant reacts at once to pain of high intensity in all states. Gerhardt et al. (1988) had shown that sound stimulation applied to the abdominal surface of sheep could result in a mean sound pressure of 135 dB, measured in utero by a hydrophone close to the fetal ear.

Responses in Fetal Compromise

Redman asked what the response was in a compromised fetus in which delivery was being considered, one which might be hypoxaemic and perhaps developing acidaemia. Such terminal circumstances were uncommon in Patrick's clinical experience in London, Ontario, and he did not answer the question directly. There are many, divergent, reports in the literature, some of which recorded no response to stimuli. Patrick and Robert Gagnon had examined 17 human fetuses at 33–40 weeks gestation with growth retardation (<10th centile), all of which had responded normally. However, in a younger group at 26–32 weeks gestation with severe growth retardation (<3rd centile), there was no response (Gagnon et al., 1988, 1989). It had taken a long time to collect this group. Much of the American literature failed to discriminate between fetuses <10th centile weight for age and sex, many of whom he regarded as within normal limits behaviourally, and those <3rd centile, which were abnormal in his view.

Visser said that the response to vibroacoustic stimuli was used in the USA as a test of neurological integrity. Yet a French group (Richards et al., 1988) had shown that anencephalic fetuses react normally. Pardi asked whether other fetal abnormalities, hydrocephalics or fetuses with chromosomal anomalies or infections had been studied. John Patrick did not know of systematic studies along these lines.

Animal Studies on Vibroacoustic Stimuli

Hanson's group in Reading had been unable to obtain fetal responses to vibroacoustic stimuli in sheep comparable to those in man. If the sheep fetus was in low-voltage electrocortical activity there was an immediate shift to high-voltage, with the onset of breathing and often some activity in the neck musculature. However, there was no comparable increase in fetal heart rate— John Patrick agreed as to the dissimilarity between these two species. The difference could not be attributed to differences in the frequency components of the stimuli, which had been explored both in London, Ontario and in Reading, England. Neither group had yet measured fetal plasma catecholamines or other hormones before or after vibroacoustic stimulation.

Both Hanson's group and that of Abrams (Abrams et al., 1987, 1989) had shown that the responses in sheep were abolished by ablation of the cochlea. Patrick said that he knew of one infant which had not responded to vibroacoustic stimuli before birth and was found to be deaf postnatally (diagnosis confirmed as deafness only). Occasionally fetal lambs did not respond, but Abrams had shown that it was possible for the sound source to be localized inappropriately on the abdomen. Challis wondered whether the position of the allantoic sac was critical, but Patrick considered that acoustic transmission through it should not be impaired. Indeed there was evidence of some concentration of sound intensity in the abdominal cavity of animals, rather than attenuation as usually anticipated.

Patrick also reported that Abrams et al. (1989) had shown that sound stimulation was associated with a large increase in O_2 metabolism (using the 2-deoxyglucose method) in the auditory pathways of fetal lambs. When the cochlea was ablated there was a great reduction in cerebral O_2 metabolism, *not* confined to the auditory pathways or their projections. The method was restricted to a single measurement per animal, so the time course of changes had not been studied.

In conclusion Dawes remarked that though no fetus had been reported as dying as a consequence of vibroacoustic stimulation, the prolonged tachycardia for up to 1 hour, so often reported, was a cause for concern; no other stimulation had caused such a response. Visser added that there were occasional more sinister changes, such as profound falls in fetal heart rate (Nijhuis et al., 1988; Scherer et al., 1988; Visser et al., 1989).

References

Abrams RM, Hutchinson AA, McTiernan MJ (1987) Am J Obstet Gynecol 157: 1438–1442.
Abrams RM, Hutchinson AA, Gerhardt KJ (1989) Dev Brain Res 48: 1–10.
Gagnon R, Hunse C, Fellows F, Carmichael L, Patrick J (1988) Am J Obstet Gynecol 158: 265–271.
Gagnon R, Hunse C, Carmichael L, Patrick J (1989) Am J Obstet Gynecol 160: 160–165.
Gerhardt KJ, Abrams RM, Kovaz BM et al. (1988) Am J Obstet Gynecol 159: 228–232.
Leader LR, Stevens AD, Lumbers ER (1988) Biol Neonat 53: 73–85.
Nijhuis JG, Kruyt N, van Wijck JAM (1988) Br J Obstet Gynaecol 95: 197–200.
Richards DS, Cefalo RC, Thorpe JM et al. (1988) Obstet Gynecol 71: 535–540.
Scherer DM, Menashe M, Sadovksy E (1988) Am J Obstet Gynecol 159: 334–335.
Van den Bergh BRH, Mulder EJH, Visser GHA et al. (1989) Early Hum Dev 19: 9–19.
Visser GHA, Mulder HH, Wit HP et al. (1989) Early Hum Dev 19: 285–296.

6

Fetal Behavioural States

D. ARDUINI AND G. RIZZO

Clinica Ostetrica e Ginecologica, Università Cattolica del Sacro Cuore, Roma, Italy

Studies on fetal lambs have shown that episodic behavioural states are already established from days 110–125 of gestation onwards (Dawes et al., 1972; Ruckebusch, 1972). The advent of ultrasound equipment allowed a non-invasive assessment of human fetal movements (Birnholz et al., 1978; Bots et al., 1981) and heart rate patterns (Evertson et al., 1979). This technical advance opened up a new field of developmental studies, which provided confirmation of results from animal models as well as evidence of new important findings. Thus Timor-Trisch et al. (1978) showed that in the human near term, fetal heart rate (FHR) and body movements (FM) are clustered in episodes resembling quiet and active phases of animal behaviour. Nijhuis et al. (1982) found evidence of stable and recurring associations between FHR, FM and fetal eye movements (FEM), similar to those used by Prechtl (1974) to identify behavioural states in the new born. These associations become particularly evident from 36 weeks of gestation onwards, permitting the identification of four different behavioural states (1F to 4F) in the human fetus.

The aim of this chapter is to report the methods used to record behavioural states, to describe their development in normal and abnormal pregnancies and to discuss the potential clinical applications of their study.

Methods

Recordings are performed on patients lying on a bed in a comfortable semi-recumbent position in a quiet room. To standardize the influences of diurnal variation and maternal food intake all the recordings are performed in the afternoon 2 hours after a standardized 1000 Kcal lunch. Three different behavioural variables, i.e. FHR, FEM and FM, are recorded simultaneously for

Fetal Autonomy and Adaptation. Edited by G. S. Dawes, A. Zacutti, F. Borruto and A. Zacutti, Jr
© 1990 John Wiley & Sons Ltd

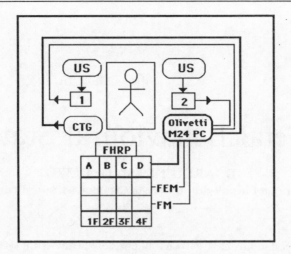

FIGURE 1 Configuration of the automatic system used for behavioural state analysis. US = ultrasound observers 1 and 2. FHRP = fetal heart rate patterns

two consecutive hours. FHR is measured by a Hewlett-Packard 8040 cardiotocograph equipped with an external ultrasound transducer. FEM and FM are determined by two observers using two real-time ultrasound instruments (Toshiba Sal 20 and Ansaldo Esacord 81) positioned to obtain a parasagittal section through the fetal face and a transverse section at the level of the upper part of the fetal abdomen respectively. In order to standardize the analysis we developed a computerized system for the acquisition and analysis of fetal behavioural states (Rizzo et al., 1988); this is based on an Olivetti M24 personal computer. As shown in Figure 1 the two observers enter individual movements in the computerized system using two remote switching devices and codified keyboards for signalling the onset and the

TABLE 1 Criteria for definition of behavioural states (FHRP = fetal heart rate patterns; FEM = fetal eye movements; FM = fetal gross body movements)

Behavioural state	FHRP*	FEM	FM
1F (quiet sleep)	A	absent	absent
2F (active sleep)	B	present	present
3F (quiet awake)	C	present	absent
4F (active awake)	D	present	present

*A = heart rate variability < 10 bpm, absence of accelerations or isolated ones.
 B = variability > 10 bpm, frequent acceleration.
 C = variability > 10 bpm, absence of accelerations.
 D = heart rate unstable with large and long-lasting accelerations.

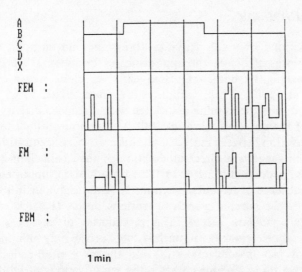

FIGURE 2 Graphic display of the behavioural variables studied as plotted by the computer. Time scale (vertical lines) = 1 minute intervals

end of each movement. Similarly they enter the periods in which a reliable view of the fetus is not obtained. FHR is taken from the RS232 port of the cardiocograph and the digitalized signal is entered into the serial port of the computer.

At the end of the recordings FHR is automatically analysed using a 3-minute moving window and divided into four different patterns (A to D) according to Nijhuis et al. (1982). An algorithm (Arduini and Rizzo, 1990) has been developed in order to differentiate the different FHR patterns. This system also computes several variables for each movement, such as the incidence, duration, lag time, % time spent moving, and these quantitative data are then related to the different FHR patterns. Finally the FHR and fetal movements are plotted on a time axis (Figure 2) and the coincidence of behavioural states are automatically calculated as in Table 1.

Development of Fetal Behavioural States

Behavioural states are clearly established by 36 weeks gestation (Nijhuis et al., 1982; Arduini et al., 1985), though the first signs of their existence are already evident by 28 weeks (Arduini et al., 1986a; Dawes, 1988) with the presence of circadian and ultradian rhythms.

Circadian Rhythms

Diurnal variations of fetal activities (breathing movements, FM, FHR) are probably present before the appearance of behavioural states and have been described in the human fetus as early as 20–22 weeks of gestation (De Vries et al., 1987). These variations are characterized by an increase of fetal activity during the evening associated with a reduced activity during the first hours of the day (Patrick et al., 1982). It is noteworthy that there is a negative correlation between maternal plasma cortisol concentrations and fetal activity, which suggests a direct modulation of fetal behaviour by maternal cortisol levels (Arduini et al., 1987b). This hypothesis is supported by studies showing the absence of circadian rhythms in fetal behaviour in patients with suppression of the adrenal glands by various means (Patrick et al., 1981; Arduini et al., 1986b, 1986c). The mechanism of action of maternal steroids on fetal behaviour is still unclear, but cortisol may modulate the fetal production of pro-opiomelanocortin, and therefore of β-endorphin, as it has been shown that naloxone causes rapid modifications of fetal behaviour (Arduini et al., 1987a).

Few data are so far available on the circadian modulation of behaviour in compromised fetuses. We recently observed the loss of the circadian rhythm of fetal activity in intrauterine growth-retarded (IUGR) fetuses, considered secondary to placental insufficiency (i.e. with abnormal Doppler velocity waveforms) as shown in Figure 3.

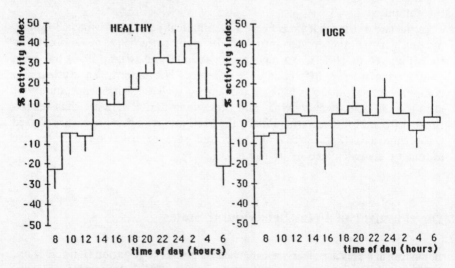

FIGURE 3 Circadian variations of fetal activity in healthy (15 cases) and intrauterine growth-retarded (IUGR) fetuses (12 cases) at 36 weeks of gestation. Data are plotted as mean values ± 1 SD

Ultradian Rhythms

Behavioural variables such as FHR, FM and FEM showed evident periodicities from 26–28 weeks gestation onwards (Arduini et al., 1986a). As fetuses grow older these variables become gradually more related temporally, and clustered, and after 36 weeks 'true' behavioural states can be detected (Nijhuis et al., 1982). The incidence of these states can be calculated before this gestational age on the basis of the proportion of coincidence between the different behavioural variables according to the criteria of Table 1. The percentage of time spent by the fetus with no coincidence in behavioural variables (% no coincidence), expressed as a function of gestational age, can be used as an index of the development of the fetal behavioural states. The reference limits of our laboratory are reported in Figure 4.

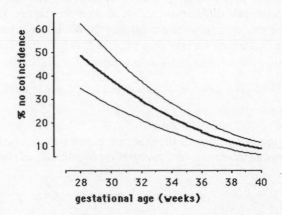

FIGURE 4   Normal ranges (mean ± 2 SD) of the proportion (%) of time in which there was no coincidence between behavioural variables constructed from 142 fetuses studied cross-sectionally

The progressive coordination of behavioural states is believed to be related to the development of the central nervous system, and several studies have shown behavioural abnormalities in compromised fetuses. In IUGR fetuses the development of behavioural states is delayed (Van Vliet et al., 1985) and these findings seem to be related to the severity of the modifications of the fetal circulation (Rizzo et al., 1987). In fetuses of type I diabetic women the coincidence of behavioural states is lower than in healthy fetuses despite optimal control of plasma glucose (Mulder et al., 1987). In hydrocephalic fetuses behavioural abnormalities are usually present and seem to be related to the severity of brain damage and neonatal outcome (Arduini et al., 1987c).

Potential Clinical Applications

Behavioural state analysis has to date been limited to research applications; to the best of our knowledge no clinical application has been reported. This is mainly due to the long observation time required for conventional analysis.

We recently reported (Arduini et al., 1989) that the study of the duration of behavioural transitions (i.e. the time intervals between two different and consecutive behavioural states) differentiates between healthy fetuses and IUGR fetuses near term. We established the normal developmental course of transitions in healthy fetuses during the third trimester of pregnancy, providing reference values for their duration and their sequence of change of behavioural variables (Arduini et al., 1990). We then compared the results of the analysis of transitions with those of conventional behavioural states, in a group of fetuses developing IUGR as predicted by abnormal Doppler velocity waveforms (Arduini et al., 1987d); we found a statistically significant correlation between the results obtained with the two different methods of analysis (Figure 5). The study of transitions allows a significant shortening of the observation time, since in our experience the first transition is evidenced after 45.4 minutes of recording (range 15–87).

Conclusions

Since the original description of the existence of behavioural states in the human fetus an increasing interest in fetal maturation has developed. Behavioural state

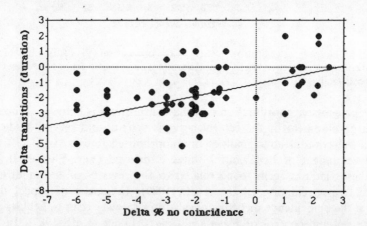

FIGURE 5   Correlation between % no coincidence and duration of transitions ($r = 0.51$, df $= 58$, $p \leq 0.001$, constant $= -1.083$, slope $= 0.383$). Data are expressed as delta values (i.e. number or fraction of standard deviation from the mean of our reference ranges)

analysis has allowed us to obtain a better knowledge of fetal physiology and to establish the normal course of development. Furthermore it has been possible to demonstrate ultradian and circadian rhythms of fetal behaviour and to clarify in part the mechanisms regulating the alternation of states. Several papers have shown abnormal behavioural patterns in sick fetuses, and the degree of abnormality seems to be related to the severity of fetal compromise.

However, behavioural state analysis has so far been limited to research applications. The use of a computerized system simplifies the acquisition of behavioural variables and shortens and standardizes analysis off-line. Finally restriction of the analysis to selected periods of fetal behaviour, such as transitions, might reduce the observation time required, make it compatible with clinical practice and provide in the near future a useful tool for fetal monitoring.

References

Arduini D and Rizzo G (1990) Quantitative analysis of fetal heart rate: its application in antepartum clinical monitoring and behavioural pattern recognition. Int J Biomed Comp 25: 247–252.

Arduini D, Rizzo G, Giorlandino C, Nava S, Dell' Acqua S, Valensise H and Romanini C (1985) The fetal behavioural states: an ultrasonic study. Prenat Diagn 5: 269–276.

Arduini D, Rizzo G, Giorlandino C, Dell' Acqua S, Valensise H, Romanini C (1986a) The development of fetal behavioural states: a longitudinal study. Prenat Diagn 6: 117–124.

Arduini D, Rizzo G, Parlati E, Giorlandino C, Valensise H, Dell' Acqua S, Romanini C (1986b) Modifications of ultradian and circadian rhythms of fetal heart rate after fetal-maternal adrenal gland suppression: a double blind study. Prenat Diagn 6: 409–417.

Arduini D, Rizzo G, Parlati E, Valensise H, Dell' Acqua S, Romanini C (1986c) Loss of circadian rhythms of fetal behaviour in a total adrenalectomized pregnant woman. Gynecol Obstet Inv 23: 226–229.

Arduini D, Rizzo G, Dell' Acqua S, Mancuso S, Romanini C (1987a) Effects of naloxone on fetal behaviour near term. Am J Obstet Gynecol 156: 474–478.

Arduini D, Rizzo G, Parlati E, Dell' Acqua S, Mancuso S, Romanini C (1987b) Are the fetal heart rate patterns related to fetal maternal endocrine rhythms at term of pregnancy? J Fetal Med 6: 53–57.

Arduini D, Rizzo G, Caforio L, Romanini C, Mancuso S (1987c) The development of behavioural states in hydrocephalic fetuses. Fetal Ther 2: 135–143.

Arduini D, Rizzo G, Romanini C, Mancuso S (1987d) Fetal blood flow velocity waveforms as predictors of growth retardation. Obstet Gynecol 70: 7–10.

Arduini D, Rizzo G, Caforio L, Boccolini MR, Romanini C, Mancuso S (1989) Behavioural state transitions in healthy and growth retarded fetuses. Early Hum Develop 19: 155–162.

Arduini D, Rizzo G, Massacesi M, Boccolini MR, Romanini C, Mancuso S (1990) Longitudinal assessment of behavioural transitions in healthy human fetuses during the last trimester of pregnancy. J Perinat Med (in press).

Birnholz JC, Stephens JC, Faria M (1978) Fetal movements patterns: a possible means of defining neurological milestones in utero. Am J Roengt 130: 537–540.

Bots RSGM, Nijhuis JG, Martin CB Jr, Prechtl HFR (1981) Human fetal eye movements: detection in utero by means of ultrasonography. Early Hum Develop 5: 87–94.

Dawes GS (1988) The development of fetal behavioural patterns. Can J Physiol Pharmacol 66: 541–548.

Dawes GS, Fox HE, Leduc BM, Liggins GC, Richards R (1972) Respiratory movements and rapid eye movement sleep in the foetal lamb. J Physiol 220: 119–143.

De Vries JIP, Visser GHA, Mulder EJH, Prechtl HFR (1987) Diurnal and other variations in fetal movements and other heart rate patterns. Early Hum Dev 15: 99–114.

Evertson LR, Gauthier RS, Schrifin BS, Paul RH (1979) Antepartum fetal heart testing. I Evolution of the non stress test. Am J Obstet Gynecol 133: 29–33.

Mulder EJH, Visser GHA, Beckedam DJ, Prechtl HFR (1987) Emergence of fetal behavioural states in fetuses of type-1 diabetic women. Early Hum Dev 15: 231–251.

Nijhuis JG, Prechtl HFR, Martin CB Jr, Bots RSGM (1982) Are there behavioural states in the human fetus? Early Hum Dev 6: 177–195.

Patrick J, Challis J, Campbell K, Carmichael L, Richardson B, Tevaarwerk G (1981) Effects of synthetic glucocorticoid on the human fetal breathing movements at 34–35 weeks gestation. Am J Obstet Gynecol 139: 324–328.

Patrick J, Campbell K, Carmichael L, Richardson B (1982) Patterns of fetal gross body movements over 24 hours observation intervals during the last 10 weeks of pregnancy. Am J Obstet Gynecol 146: 363–371.

Prechtl HFR (1974) The behavioural states of newborn infants (a review). Brain Res 76: 185–212.

Rizzo G, Arduini D, Pennestrì F, Romanini C, Mancuso S (1987) The fetal behaviour in growth retardation: its relationships to fetal blood flow. Prenat Diagn 7: 229–238.

Rizzo G, Arduini D, Romanini C, Mancuso S (1988) Computer-assisted analysis of fetal behavioural states. Prenat Diagn 8: 479–484.

Ruckebush Y (1972) Development of sleep and wakefulness in the foetal lamb. Electro-encephalograph. Clin Neurophysiol 32: 119–128.

Timor-Trisch IE, Dierker LJ, Hertz RH, Deagan NC, Rosen MG (1978) Studies of antepartum behavioural state in the human fetus at term. Am J Obstet Gynecol 132: 524–528.

Van Vliet MAT, Martin CB Jr, Nijhuis JG, Prechtl HFR (1985) Behavioural states in growth retarded fetuses. Early Hum Dev 12: 183–197.

Discussion

Difficulties in Identifying Behavioural States

Dawes was concerned whether the attenuation of FHR variation and of fetal movements in intrauterine growth retardation might have caused difficulties in applying the criteria used to identify fetal states, which had been adopted in Holland from observations on healthy vigorous fetuses. Growth-retarded fetuses continued to show episodic activity but at a reduced amplitude; it was then more difficult to be certain of the end-points. Patrick recalled the observations of Dennis Worthington et al. (1981), who had shown that in growth-retarded sheep (the progeny of ewes in which many uterine caruncles were cauterized to limit development of the placentomes) the incidence of fetal breathing movements was halved. Fetal breathing continued, but greatly reduced.

Patrick asked what was responsible for the 350 s gap between states 1F and 2F in man. What variables were missing to provide the designation of a transitional stage? Rizzo replied that *in the normal fetus*, studied longitudinally from 28 weeks gestational age, there was at first no prominent, leading variable whose appearance or disappearance heralded the transition. As age increased the fetal body movements changed first, to be followed by changes in eye movements, breathing, and FHR variation (Arduini et al., 1990). *In the growth-retarded fetus* the sequence remained disorganized at a comparable age.

Patrick then drew attention to the fact that in sheep the transition between states, analogous to quiet or rapid-eye-movement postnatally, had conventionally been identified by the change from low- to high-voltage electrocortical activity, or vice versa. Hazel Szeto (personal communication) had recently used a method developed by anaesthetists, defining the point at which 90% of the spectral power (of the electrocorticogram) had been identified in a transition; she thus defined four states, two of which usually occurred *between* episodes of low- and high-voltage activity. He also drew attention to the difficulties arising where variables conventionally used as criteria of fetal sleep states were independently regulated by physiological changes. When the fetus was made mildly hypoxic, some such variables (e.g. breathing or limb movements) could fail to appear even when the electrocortical activity became characteristic of rapid-eye-movement sleep.

Rizzo agreed that under several clinical conditions, growth retardation, maternal diabetes and fetal hydrocephaly or hypoxaemia, several research groups had observed a disturbance of transitional states. The effects could be non-specific, but he did not categorize particular features.

Abnormalities of Function or Brain Development

Pardi thought that abnormalities of brain development, such as anencephaly, should provide good material in which to study aberrations of behavioural states. Rizzo had found such disturbances, in transition between behavioural states, in hydrocephaly but had no experience in anencephaly. In hydrocephaly the severity of the behavioural changes was a good indicator of the prognosis (Arduini et al., 1982). Visser quoted the work of Terao et al. (1984) in which it was reported that when the hindbrain was absent in anencephaly there was no behavioural cycling. And he mentioned that a persistent flat FHR pattern had been seen after antenatal fetal decerebration (Dijxhoorn et al., 1986, Visser, 1988).

Rizzo referred to studies by Visser and his colleagues in Groningen on the fetuses of diabetic mothers. Visser stated that these abnormalities in state transition were not related to the degree of maternal diabetic control. They occurred even when the mother was well controlled and were also present directly after birth. At follow-up (1.5–4 years) psychomotor development was normal, suggesting that the abnormal development of behaviour was likely to be due to the altered intrauterine environment. In reply to Pardi, Visser said that this phenomenon in diabetes was the subject of research; it had not been allowed to influence clinical decisions in the management of diabetic pregnancy.

Dawes said that large lesions had been made in the brains of fetal lambs, such as transection rostrally through the hypothalamus, with no gross change in normal fetal behaviour, in electrocorticographic activity or episodic breathing movements (Dawes et al., 1983). The damage had to be more caudal, in the lower brainstem, pons or medulla, to cause an overt change in behaviour. There was no convincing evidence of a disruption of sleep state associated with progressive deterioration leading to death, other than the attentuation of electrocortical activity before death from hypoxia.

Doppler Flow Studies

Mandruzzato then widened the discussion to consider the changes in flow velocity waveforms in human growth retardation. He considered, in contradiction to Lin and Evans (1984) that abnormalities in the FHR, and especially in FHR variation, occurred as early as 'were as precocious as', and were related to abnormal Doppler flow velocity waveform findings, when the evaluation of the CTG is performed by computer analysis, as for instance the system developed by Dawes, which he was using. Abnormalities observed in traditional ways only became apparent days or weeks after abnormal Doppler findings in cases with IUGR. There was no point in measuring one clinical test against another, when no one know which, if either, gave reliable results. In a recent meeting in Barcelona (European Committee for Doppler Technology in Perinatal Medicine; 27–29 September 1989) there was a consensus view that the predictive accuracy of Doppler screening of maternal or fetal vessels was poor. It was of use in predicting the subsequent development of fetal distress in cases *already recognized* as being growth retarded, i.e. in a selected high-risk population.

Rizzo had no experience with Doppler ultrasound in a low-risk population. He had applied this technique in a high-risk population, and his results (Arduini et al., 1987a, 1987b) were in agreement with the literature, suggesting a role in the prediction of hypertension, fetal distress and IUGR (Campbell et al., 1986; Trudinger et al., 1987; Steel et al., 1988). Schulman (1989) had also recently demonstrated its efficacy in a low-risk population. In his experience Doppler abnormalities precede FHR abnormalities (Arduini, 1989a) as also shown by the literature (Trudinger, 1987; Laurin, 1987; and by Visser in the following chapter). Several studies had demonstrated a close correlation between fetal pO_2 or oxygen content, measured at cordocentesis or after caesarean section, and changes in Doppler velocity waveforms recorded from different fetal vessels, including the descending aorta (Soothill et al., 1986), umbilical artery (Ferrazzi, 1988), and internal carotid artery (Arduini, 1989b).

Behavioural States

In conclusion Dawes pointed out that in both sheep and man the gradual development of fetal behavioural states was spread over several weeks—from 28 to 36 weeks in man—so that for a large part of the time when clinical decisions might have to be taken on grounds of deteriorating fetal health, the so-called state-related variables were discordant or unreliable. So was the definition of fetal states of clinical use? In reply Rizzo said that the definition of behavioural state in the fetus required 2 hours of study, and on that ground could not be used as a routine clinical tool. Identification of a transitional episode could be achieved more rapidly, in less than an hour. Yet at the present its importance still lay in advancing physiological knowledge as a background to practice.

References

Arduini D (1989a) Br Med J 298: 1561–1562.
Arduini D (1989b) Gynecol Obstet Inv 27: 183–187.
Arduini D et al. (1982) Fetal Ther 2: 135–143.
Arduini D et al. (1987a) Obstet Gynecol 70: 7–10.
Arduini D et al. (1987b) Eur J Obstet Gynecol Reprod Biol 26: 335–341.
Arduini D et al. (1989a) Early Hum Dev 18: 155–162.
Arduini D et al. (1990) J. Perinatal Med (in press).
Campbell S et al. (1986) Obstet Gynecol 68: 649–653.
Dawes GS, Gardner WN, Johnston BM, Walker DW (1983) J Physiol 335: 535–553.
Dijxhoorn MJ, Visser GHA, Fidler VJ et al. (1986) Br J Obstet Gynaecol 93: 217–222.
Ferrazzi E et al. (1988) Am J Obstet Gynecol 159: 1081–1087.
Laurin J et al. (1987) Br J Obstet Gynaecol 94: 940.
Lin CC and Evans MI (1984) Intrauterine Growth Retardation: Pathophysiology and Clinical Management. McGraw Hill, New York.
Schulman H et al. (1989) Am J Obstet Gynecol 160: 192–196.
Soothill PN et al. (1986) Lancet ii: 1118–1120.
Steel SA et al. (1988) Eur J Obstet Gynecol Reprod Biol 28: 279–287.
Terao T, Kawashima Y, Noto H et al. (1984) Am J Obstet Gynec 149: 201–208.
Trudinger BJ (1987) Br J Obstet Gynaecol 93: 171.
Trudinger BJ, Cook CM, Giles WB et al. (1987) Lancet i: 188–190.
Visser GHA (1988) Baillière's Clin Obstet Gynaecol 2:117–124.
Worthington D, Piercy WN, Smith BJ (1981) Obstet Gynecol 58: 215–221.

7

Serial Observations on Adaptation in the Human Fetus

G. H. A. VISSER AND D. J. BEKEDAM

Department of Obstetrics and Gynaecology, State University, Groningen,
The Netherlands

With progressive deterioration of the fetal condition several changes occur in fetal motor patterns and behaviour and in the cardiovascular system. Most of these changes have only been studied cross-sectionally and data relating them to the actual fetal condition are scarce. Nevertheless gradually a picture has developed of when changes in heart rate and movement patterns occur with progressive deterioration.

In this paper these changes are rank ordered, and related to the actual fetal condition and (where possible) to neurological outcome. For reasons of simplicity data are restricted to intrauterine growth retarded (IUGR) fetuses; specifically those small-for-dates fetuses in which growth restriction is likely to be due to an impaired utero-placental circulation, with consequent fetal malnutrition.

Adaptation implies a modification that makes the fetus better suited to survive (intact) in utero. It will be demonstrated that some changes in fetal behaviour and in the cardiovascular system can indeed be considered as signs of adaptation. Others are indications of disturbances in function, which may result in organ damage.

Heart Rate and Movement Patterns in IUGR Fetuses

Murata et al. (1982) found that with progressive deterioration in fetal condition in the rhesus monkey, late decelerations of the fetal heart rate appeared first. This condition was associated with fetal hypoxaemia. The incidence of accelerations (and possibly of movements) decreased later, when the pH also

Fetal Autonomy and Adaptation. Edited by G. S. Dawes, A. Zacutti, F. Borruto and A. Zacutti, Jr
© 1990 John Wiley & Sons Ltd

fell. In growth-retarded fetal sheep it has been shown that chronic hypoxaemia (and hypoglycaemia) sometimes can be present for weeks before acidaemia and finally intrauterine death occurs (Robinson et al., 1985).

There is evidence that changes in heart rate (and movement) patterns in the growth-retarded human fetus follow more or less the same pattern as found in the rhesus monkey. A possible rank order, in which these changes occur with progressive deterioration of the fetal condition is shown in Figure 1. Centrally placed in this figure is the occurrence of late heart rate decelerations. The suggested rank order is based on the following studies.

In IUGR fetuses with a decelerative fetal heart rate pattern umbilical artery pO_2 values obtained at elective (primary) caesarean section have been found to be significantly lower than those in a control group or in IUGR fetuses with a normal heart rate pattern (Bekedam et al., 1987). No differences were found in pH values, indicating that in IUGR fetuses antenatal heart rate decelerations are associated with hypoxaemia and not with acidaemia. Recently this has been confirmed by comparing antepartum heart rate records to fetal blood gases, obtained at cordocentesis. In 41 out of the 45 small-for-gestational age fetuses with a normal ('reactive') heart rate pattern, pO_2 values were normal, whereas acidaemia was absent in all 45 cases. In the presence of late decelerations, however, 12 out of the 13 fetuses were hypoxaemic and/or mildly acidaemic (Visser et al., 1989).

Using a numerical analysis it has been shown that in IUGR fetuses long-term heart rate variation is usually low. However, in the absence of decelerations this variation is nearly always within the (lower) normal range (Visser, 1984). On the other hand, when late decelerations are present heart rate variation is

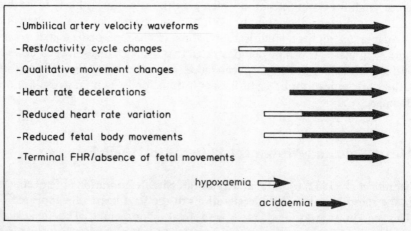

FIGURE 1   Suggested rank ordering in which blood velocity waveforms, movements and heart rate changes occur in growth-retarded human fetuses with progressive deterioration of the fetal condition. Redrawn from Visser et al., 1990

further (abnormally) reduced in the majority of cases (Bekedam et al., 1987). This implies that in general the heart rate variation pattern of growth-retarded fetuses cannot be distinguished from that of normal ones before late decelerations appear, and, consequently, that a reduction of long-term heart rate variation has to be considered as a rather late sign of fetal compromise. Recently we could confirm this in a longitudinal study of 13 growth-retarded fetuses (Snijders et al., 1988) in whom heart rate records were analysed using an on-line computer system (Dawes et al., 1985). With time there was a gradual fall in heart rate variation and on average variation fell below the norm (= 30 msec) at the same time as decelerations occurred (Figure 2). There were, however, large interfetal differences: in some fetuses a reduced variation preceded the occurrence of decelerations by weeks, whereas in others variation fell only after the occurrence of decelerations.

In a study in which the different components of the FHR pattern (accelerations, baseline variation, decelerations) were related to data obtained at cordocentesis, the negative and positive predictive values for fetal hypoxaemia and/or acidaemia were almost the same (81 to 88% and 63 to 89%, respectively) (Visser et al., 1989). This also suggests that with progressive deterioration of the fetal condition, changes in these components occur approximately at the same time. More or less similar findings were made by Van der Slikke (1981). He analysed fetal heart rate patterns visually in 13 growth-retarded fetuses 3 to 12 days before intrauterine death. Heart rate decelerations occurred at the same time as the FHR band width decreased and accelerations disappeared.

It has been shown that long-term heart rate variation is reduced before fetal acidaemia develops (Henson et al., 1983). The initial reduction in heart rate

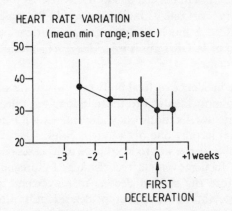

FIGURE 2   Changes in long-term heart rate variation (mean 1-minute range; in msec) in a longitudinal study in 13 growth-retarded fetuses (median and interquartile ranges). The data are grouped according to the first occurrence of late decelerations. The lower range of normality is 30 msec. From Visser et al., 1990

variation is, therefore, not caused by fetal acidaemia. Hypoxaemia, on the other hand, may play a role, as variation decreases below the normal range with the appearance of heart rate decelerations. Furthermore, significant correlations between heart rate variation ('mean-one-minute range') and pO_2 values as obtained at elective caesarean section or at cordocentesis have been found ($r = 0.52$ and 0.48, respectively) (Smith et al., 1988; Ribbert et al., 1989). The temporary decrease in heart rate variation directly after 'hypoxaemic' events (late decelerations) and the increase during maternal hyperoxygenation also indicate the relationship of variation with the oxygenation status of the fetus (Bekedam and Visser, 1985; Bekedam, 1989). These data indicate that antepartum late heart rate decelerations and a decrease of heart rate variation coincide with the occurrence of fetal hypoxaemia. The lack of identification of fetuses with a pO_2 in the lower normal range indicates that antepartum FHR monitoring is not a reliable screening method for a forthcoming impairment.

Late and (prolonged) variable decelerations are easy to assess visually. This does not hold for heart rate variation. The advantages of an objective numerical analysis of heart rate variation include:

1. Identification of fetuses in which a reduced variation precedes the occurrence of decelerations or in which decelerations do not occur during each record.
2. Precision of the degree of impairment in fetuses with late heart rate decelerations present; this is especially important at early gestation when further maturation in utero might be considered.
3. Following longitudinally variation in fetuses thought to be at risk of impairment. Both in normal and in IUGR fetuses there are large interfetal differences in heart rate variation, but within the same individual variation remains within a much narrower range (Snijders et al., 1988). In the surveillance of IUGR fetuses it is, therefore, advisable to use each fetus as its own control.

Changes in the incidence of fetal body movements (as observed by real-time ultrasound) are almost identical to those in long-term heart rate variation. In the absence of late decelerations body movements fell below the norm ($= 5\%$ of recording time) in only one out of eight cases, whereas in the presence of decelerations this incidence was reduced in 18 of 27 cases (Bekedam et al., 1987). From subjective fetal movement records kept by pregnant women it is also known that, before the sudden decline in movements which may indicate impending fetal death, the movement incidence is still within the normal range (Sadovsky et al., 1974; Pearson and Weaver, 1976). So a decline in the incidence of fetal movements must also be considered a late sign of fetal deterioration. The assumption that a decrease in movements is associated with hypoxaemia is supported by the temporary decrease in incidence of generalized body movements and of breathing movements during and directly after 'hypoxaemic' events and by the increase during maternal hyperoxygenation (Bekedam and Visser, 1985; Bekedam, 1989; Ruedrick et al., 1989).

In fetal sheep also acute hypoxaemia is associated with a reduction in breathing and other movements (Natale et al., 1981; Bocking and Harding, 1986). The decrease in limb and body movements cannot be explained by an increase in the percentage of time that fetuses spend in high-voltage electrocortical activity, since in fetal sheep these movements tend to be more numerous during high-voltage activity (Natale et al., 1981).

With further deterioration of the fetal condition movements disappear and the fetal heart rate pattern becomes 'terminal': heart rate variation is greatly reduced (not measurable visually) and there are repeated late, mostly shallow, decelerations. This condition is strongly associated with fetal acidaemia and, at elective caesarean section, a pH in the umbilical artery of less than 7.15 has been found in the majority of cases (Visser et al., 1980). If delivery does not occur in due course, fetal death will occur within one week.

Fetal heart rate and movement changes that precede the occurrence of late decelerations are, in general, more difficult to quantify. From subjective records kept by the women it is known that, sometimes weeks before movements decline, an increase in the percentage of weak movements occurs, with a decrease of strong and 'rolling' movements (Sadovsky et al., 1979). Using real-time ultrasound, slow monotonous movements of small amplitude can be observed. Although techniques for quantification have been developed, objective assessment of these changes remains difficult. For the ultrasonographer familiar with normal fetal motility these changes are, however, usually evident; in a series in which we investigated this a high inter-observer agreement was found (Bekedam et al., 1985). Manning et al. (1981), who developed a biophysical profile score, assessed the quality of motility by observing limb movements. In normal fetuses, following extension of a limb, a rapid return to flexion can be observed, whereas in compromised fetuses this does not occur.

A disturbance in the development of fetal behavioural states also precedes the occurrence of late decelerations. From 36–38 weeks onwards, the normal fetus exhibits well-regulated fetal behavioural states with simultaneous changes in heart rate, eye movement and gross body movement patterns (Nijhuis et al., 1982) This is in contrast to growth-retarded term fetuses in whom a disturbance in behavioural state development has been described; especially, the inability to synchronize the state variables at the transitions was evident (Van Vliet et al., 1985; Arduini et al., 1989). As the fetuses from these studies had normal heart rate records, it is likely that impaired development of behavioural states precedes the occurrence of heart rate decelerations, just as qualitative changes in fetal motility do.

Doppler Blood Flow Velocity Waveform Patterns

Earlier signs of fetal impairment may be detected by Doppler recordings of umbilical artery blood flow waveform patterns. Changes in these patterns are thought to indicate increased vascular placental resistance. However, other explanations for the changes in waveform patterns, such as an increase in blood viscosity or reduced arterial blood pressure, have not been excluded, as most studies have concerned the 'inaccessible' human fetus.

Reuwer et al. (1987) found abnormal waveform patterns of the umbilical artery at least 9 days prior to the occurrence of heart rate decelerations. In 29 IUGR fetuses that we followed longitudinally the median duration of the interval between the first abnormal waveform pattern of the umbilical artery and the first antepartum heart rate deceleration was 17 days (Bekedam, 1989). Thus, in IUGR fetuses in general abnormal umbilical artery waveform patterns preceded the occurrence of antepartum decelerations by several weeks. Between fetuses the duration of this time interval differs considerably (0–60 days!) and occasionally decelerations occur when Doppler recordings are still normal (Bekedam, 1989). This indicates that normal umbilical artery waveform patterns cannot be considered as definitive proof of fetal well-being and that Doppler recordings are of limited value as to the timing of delivery. Abnormal Doppler recordings are, however, a strict indication for intensive (fetal heart rate) monitoring.

In growth-retarded fetuses a relative increase of diastolic blood flow velocities has been described in the internal carotid artery (Wladimiroff et al., 1986; Arduini et al., 1988). This phenomenon might reflect a decreased vascular resistance in the fetal cerebrum and a redistribution of cardiac output in favour of the brain, i.e. a 'brain sparing' effect. It is unknown at what stage of uteroplacental impairment this occurs. Own experience suggests that with more or less acute hypoxaemia Doppler waveform changes in the carotid precede those in the umbilical artery.

Adaptation or Organ Damage?

Fetal movements consume significant amounts of oxygen. In fetal sheep oxygen consumption fell by 17% after neuromuscular blockade. (Rurak and Gruber, 1983) and pO_2 values rose by a similar percentage (Nathanielsz et al., 1982; Rurak and Gruber, 1983). Reduction of fetal movements when oxygen supply is limited therefore aids in maximizing delivery of oxygen to vital organs. Such a reduction can be considered as adaptation. The same holds for redistribution of blood to organs such as the heart and brain. Redistribution has been demonstrated to occur in hypoxaemic conditions in fetal sheep (Peeters et al., 1979; Goetzman et al., 1984). In human IUGR fetuses redistribution of blood in favour of the brain has been suggested by blood flow velocity waveform studies (Wladimiroff et al., 1986; Arduini et al., 1988). Both in humans and in sheep this adaptation can be reversed by maternal hyperoxygenation (Goetzman et al., 1984; Arduini et al., 1988).

The usefulness of reduction of movements and of blood flow redistribution has been demonstrated nicely by an experiment in which oxygen was administered to women carrying an IUGR fetus (Bekedam, 1989). During hyperoxygenation fetal movements and heart rate variation increased. However, after discontinuation of oxygen there was a temporary impairment of the fetal heart rate pattern with an increase of heart rate decelerations. The increase in movements (and oxygen demand) and possibly a reversal of blood redistribution are likely to have caused this impairment. In the clinical situation this implies that when oxygen administration is considered as a 'treatment', it should be administered continuously without interruption.

Movements and heart rate accelerations are linked together. A reduction in the size and number of accelerations—and, therefore, of heart rate variation—as a consequence of a reduction of fetal movements, fits the concept of adaptation. It is hard, however, to consider the occurrence of late heart rate decelerations as a sign of adaptation. It is more likely that they are just signs of fetal hypoxaemia. There are only a few studies concerning the relationship between antepartum heart rate abnormalities and neurological outcome. In all, however, a definite relationship between heart rate decelerations and neurological morbidity was found (see Visser, 1988). This stresses the impact of prenatal hypoxaemia on brain development. In IUGR fetuses hypoxaemia is probably associated with chronic hypoglycaemia (Robinson et al., 1985; Soothill et al., 1987) and deprivation of other nutrients. In these fetuses brain damage is, therefore, more likely to be due to chronic malnutrition (including hypoxaemia), rather than simply to hypoxaemia. This reasoning can to a large extent be supported by the morphological findings in human IUGR fetuses (Dobbing, 1974) and in animal models (Bedi, 1984), where a smaller brain size, fewer cells, deficits in synapse-to-neurone ratios and reduced dendritic growth are found, rather than distinct localized lesions. The latter are often found after (acute) asphyxia (Kreusser and Volpe, 1984). In IUGR fetuses the occurrence of antepartum decelerations might be considered as a sign of chronic malnutrition, a sign related to impaired brain development.

The abnormal quality of fetal movements and the disturbance in the development of behavioural states are also likely to be indicators of impaired development, rather than signs of adaptation. They occur already before the development of evident hypoxaemia and have also been described in growth-retarded newborn infants in whom the metabolic state was restored and adequate (Michaelis et al., 1971; Schulte et al., 1971). This suggests that impairment of neurological development occurs before hypoxaemia develops.

Concluding Remarks

In this paper a possible rank order is presented of changes in fetal heart rate patterns, body movements and Doppler waveform patterns of the umbilical artery, which occur with progressive deterioration of the fetal condition. The data are restricted to IUGR fetuses and do not apply to a whole population. The predictive value of late heart rate decelerations appears higher in IUGR fetuses than in ones which are normally grown (Visser et al., 1980). The rank order might be of help in the understanding of changes which occur under pathophysiological conditions. It might also be helpful in establishing the diagnostic value of the various assessment techniques, of assessing effects of treatment modalities and of determining the timing of delivery of the IUGR fetus. As to the latter there are, however, still many uncertainties. In general, growth-retarded fetuses should be delivered before signs of hypoxaemia occur. Yet, as indicated above, this will not solve all the problems. Moreover, delivery at an earlier age might increase other (neonatal) risks. Research directed towards the prevention of growth retardation would seem to hold more promise with respect to the prevention of neurological handicaps than further refinement of the assessment techniques for studying the fetal condition.

References

Arduini D, Rizzo G, Mancuso S, Romanini C (1988) Short-term effects of maternal oxygen administration on blood flow velocity waveforms in healthy and growth-retarded fetuses. Am J Obstet Gynecol 159: 1077–1080.

Arduini D, Rizzo G, Caforio L, Boccolini MR, Romanini C, Mancuso S (1989) Behavioural state transitions in healthy and growth retarded fetuses. Early Hum Dev 19: 155.

Bedi KS (1984) Effects of undernutrition on brain morphology: A critical review of methods and results. In: Current Topics in Research on Synapses 2: 93–163, Alan R. Liss, New York.

Bekedam DJ (1989) Fetal heart rate and movement patterns in growth retardation. Ph.D. Thesis, University of Groningen.

Bekedam DJ and Visser GHA (1985) Effects of hypoxemic events on breathing, body movements and heart rate variation. A study in growth retarded human fetuses. Am J Obstet Gynecol, 153: 52–56.

Bekedam DJ, Visser GHA, de Vries JJ, Prechtl HFR (1985) Motor behaviour in the growth retarded fetus. Early Hum Dev 12: 155–165.

Bekedam DJ, Visser GHA, Mulder EJH, Poelmann-Weesjes G (1987) Heart rate variation and movement incidence in growth-retarded fetuses: the significance of antenatal late heart rate decelerations. Am J Obstet Gynecol 157: 126–133.

Bocking AD and Harding R (1986) Effects of reduced uterine blood flow on electrocortical activity, breathing, and skeletal muscle activity in fetal sheep. Am J Obstet Gynecol 154: 655–660.

Dawes GS, Redman CWG, Smith JH (1985) Improvement in the registration and analysis of fetal heart rate records at the bedside. Br J Obstet Gynaecol 92: 317–325.

Dobbing J (1974) The later development of the brain and its vulnerability. In: Scientific Foundations of Paediatrics (Eds: Davis JA and Dobbing J), pp 565–587. Heinemann, London.

Goetzman BW, Itskovitz J, Rudolph AM (1984) Fetal adaptations to spontaneous hypoxemia and responses to maternal oxygen breathing. Biol Neonate 46: 276–284.

Henson GL, Dawes GS, Redman CWG (1983) Antenatal fetal heart-rate variability in relation to fetal acid-base status at Caesarean section. Br J Obstet Gynaecol 90: 516–521.

Kreusser KL and Volpe JJ (1984) The neurological outcome of perinatal asphyxia. In: Early Brain Damage, Vol 1 (Eds: Almli CR and Finger S), pp 151–168. Academic Press, Orlando.

Manning FA, Baskett TF, Morrison I, Lange I (1981) Fetal biophysical profile scoring: a prospective study in 1184 high-risk patients. Am J Obstet Gynecol 140: 289–294.

Michaelis R, Schulte FJ, Nolte R (1971) Motor-behaviour of small for gestational infants. J Pediatr 76: 208.

Murata Y, Martin CB, Ikenone T et al. (1982) Fetal heart rate accelerations and late decelerations during the course of intrauterine death in chronically catheterized rhesus monkeys. Am J Obstet Gynecol 144: 218–223.

Natale R, Clewlow F, Dawes GS (1981) Measurement of fetal forelimb movements in the lamb in utero. Am J Obstet Gynecol 140: 545–551.

Nathanielsz PW, Yu HK, Calabum TC (1982) Effect of abolition on fetal movement on intravascular pO_2 and incidence of tonic myometrial contractures in the pregnant ewe at 114 to 134 days' gestation. Am J Obstet Gynecol 144: 614–618.

Nijhuis JG, Prechtl HFR, Martin CB Jr, Bots RSGM (1982) Are there any behavioural states in the human fetus? Early Hum Dev 6: 177.

Pearson JF and Weaver JB (1976) Fetal activity and fetal well-being: an evaluation. Br Med J i: 1305–1307.

Peeters LLH, Sheldon RE, Jones MD, Makowski EI, Meschia G (1979) Blood flow to fetal organs as a function of arterial oxygen content. Am J Obstet Gynecol 135: 637–643.

Reuwer PJHM, Sijmons EA, Rietman GW et al (1987) Intrauterine growth retardation: prediction of perinatal distress by Doppler ultrasound. Lancet ii: 415–418.

Ribbert LSM, Nicolaides KH, Visser GHA (1989) Correlation between computerized fetal heart rate data and blood gases obtained by cordocentesis: a study in 19 growth retarded fetuses. Abstracts 16th meeting of the Society for the Study of Fetal Physiology, University of Reading, F9.

Robinson JS, Falconer J, Owens JA (1985) Influence of growth retardation on functional capacity of fetal organ systems. In: Preterm Labour and its Consequences (Eds: Beard RW and Sharp F), pp 39–52. The Royal College of Obstetricians and Gynaecologists, London.

Ruedrick DA, Devoe LD, Searle N (1989) Effects of maternal hyperoxia on the biophysical assessment of fetuses with suspected intrauterine growth retardation. Am J Obstet Gynecol 161: 188–192.

Rurak DW and Gruber NC (1983) Effect of neuromuscular blockade on oxygen consumption and blood gases in the fetal lamb. Am J Obstet Gynecol 145: 258–262.

Sadovsky E, Yaffe H, Polishuk WZ (1974) Fetal movement monitoring in normal and pathologic pregnancy. Int J Gynaecol Obstet 12: 75–79.

Sadovsky E, Laufer N, Allen JW (1979) The incidence of different types of fetal movements during pregnancy. Br J Obstet Gynaecol 86: 10–14.

Schulte FJ, Schremf G, Hinze G (1971) Maternal toxemia, fetal malnutrition and motor behaviour in the newborn. Pediatrics 48: 871.

Smith JH, Anand KJS, Cotes PM et al. (1988) Antenatal fetal heart rate variation in relation to the respiratory and metabolic status of the compromised human fetus. Br J Obstet Gynaecol 95: 980.

Snijders RJM, Ribbert LSM, Franssens M, Visser GHA (1989) Heart rate variability in small-for-dates fetuses with abnormal umbilical artery velocity wave forms. Abstracts

3rd International Conference on Fetal and Neonatal Physiological Measurements (Ed: Marsal K), p 87. Ronneby, Sweden.

Soothill PW, Nicolaides KH, Campbell S (1987) Prenatal asphyxia, hyperlacticaemia, hypoglycaemia and erythroblastosis in growth retarded fetuses. Br Med J 294: 1051–1053.

Van der Slikke JW (1981) Antepartum Cardiotocografie. Ph.D. Thesis, University of Amsterdam.

Van Vliet MAT, Martin CB, Nijhuis JG, Prechtl HFR (1985) Behavioural states in the growth retarded human fetus. Early Hum Dev 12: 183–198.

Visser GHA (1984) Antenatal cardiotocography in the evaluation of fetal well-being. Austr NZ J Obstet Gynecol 24: 80–85.

Visser GHA (1988) Abnormal antepartum fetal heart rate patterns and subsequent handicap. In: Antenatal and Perinatal Causes of Handicap: Baillière's Clin Obstet Gynaecol 2/1: 117–124.

Visser GHA, Bekedam DJ, Ribbert LSM (1990) Changes in antepartum heart rate patterns with progressive deterioration of the fetal condition. Int J Biomed Comput 25: 239–246.

Visser GHA, Redman CWG, Huisjes HJ, Turnbull AC (1980) Nonstressed antepartum heart rate monitoring: implications of decelerations after spontaneous contractions. Am J Obstet Gynecol 138: 429–435.

Visser GHA, Sadovsky G, Nicolaides KH (1990) Antepartum heart rate patterns in small for gestational age third trimester fetuses: correlations with blood gases obtained at cordocentesis. Am J Obstet Gynecol 162: 698–703.

Wladimiroff JW, Tonge HM, Stewart PA (1986) Doppler ultrasound assessment of cerebral blood flow in the human fetus. Br J Obstet Gynaecol 93: 471.

Discussion

Diagnosis and Treatment of Fetal Deterioration

In reply to a question as to what factors should be taken into account, in deciding on delivery of a growth-retarded fetus at 27 weeks, Visser said that in early gestation the prognosis is mainly determined by the gestational age at birth (Yu et al., 1986). At this age, growth-retarded fetuses should, therefore, be left in utero as long as possible and only be delivered when acidaemia and impending death are thought to be likely. With abnormal flow velocity waveform patterns and the occurrence of heart rate decelerations, pregnancy might still be continued, provided heart rate variation and fetal movements are not greatly reduced. A reduction of long-term FHR variation below 15 msec (mean minute range; as analysed numerically) or a dramatic decrease of fetal movements (below ± 4% of recording time as observed by real-time ultrasound) were in his opinion indications for operative delivery. Much depends on the speed of decline in FHR variation, which could give a safety margin of as little as 1–3 days or as much as 4 weeks. Patrick pointed out that a flat FHR (gross reduction of FHR variation) antenatally, *without fetal acidaemia*, might indicate the use of drugs or the presence of severe brain anomalies or damage. If there were no facilities for computerized measurement of FHR variation some care had to be taken, for visual analysis was more difficult at 27–29 weeks gestation than at 31–33 weeks.

As to the timing of delivery of the growth-retarded fetus Visser thought that there were more uncertainties at 30 or 32 weeks gestation. For instance, in the presence of abnormal flow velocity waveform patterns and reduced heart rate variation, was it better to deliver the fetus or to increase maturation further in utero? Visser said that there really should be a controlled trial to solve this issue!

Early in gestation some time might be gained in utero by hyperoxygenation of the pregnant woman with 50% O_2 continuously (Nicolaides et al., 1987). Visser had treated some women with fetal growth retardation with this 'therapy' and had found an increase of both long-term FHR variation and fetal movements (unpublished observations). However, after an initial increase these variables decreased at the same rate as before. After approximately 7 days the values were identical to those before hyperoxygenation and it became necessary to deliver the fetus by caesarean section. The problem with this form of treatment, of fetuses whose growth-retardation is due to placental insufficiency, is that it does not provide additional nutrients, only oxygen. The only possible benefit is greater maturation in utero.

Redman asked whether Visser was sufficiently confident of the benefits of maternal hyperoxygenation to recommend it for general use, or should there be a randomized trial? Visser thought it beneficial but agreed that a trial was necessary to measure both the risks and the benefits. Ellendorff emphasized the risks of high oxygen pressures, but Visser replied that the data from Nicolaides et al. (1987) showed that the fetal p_aO_2 was not increased to dangerous levels (not above 35 mmHg). Thornburg raised the question of whether even this rise might not cause cerebral vascular constriction in the fetus. Visser said that Arduini et al. (1988) had shown that there is usually a low resistance in blood flow to the brain of growth-retarded fetuses, as shown by Doppler waveform patterns. Maternal hyperoxygenation increases 'resistance' to the normal range, 'resistance' in the descending aorta decreases simultaneously. He added that when in such cases maternal O_2 administration is interrupted or concluded, sometimes large decelerations appear, perhaps as a consequence of a reversed redistribution of cardiac output. Thornburg was concerned that both Blanco et al. (1988) and Teitel (1988) had found severe placental vasoconstriction on raising fetal p_aO_2 by ventilating a lamb in utero with O_2-enriched air. Yet both Rizzo and Visser were sure that there was short-term fetal improvement, with better FHR patterns and more sustained fetal movements, on maternal oxygen administration. It was, however, not yet certain whether an encouraging positive response was diagnostic of severe deterioration; nor whether failure to respond was evidence of a terminal condition or of a normal fetus. This was an additional argument for a proper trial.

In reply to a question as to what diagnostic emphasis he put on the appearance of decelerations, in addition to reduced FHR variation, Visser said that he took both into account. The presence of decelerations was most likely associated with, perhaps, a transient episode of hypoxaemia. If recurrent late decelerations were present at 26–28 weeks it was nevertheless sometimes possible to wait a few weeks before delivery, provided fetal movements continued and were vigorous and with good FHR variation. At 32–33 weeks he would deliver by section, because further risk was not justified; the probability of satisfactory neonatal survival was then good.

Rizzo enquired about the significance of late or variable decelerations in these circumstances. Visser replied that there were often no discernible pre-labour (Braxton-Hicks) uterine contractions discernible, by which such decelerations could be recognized. If the shape of the deceleration resembled that of an inverted uterine contraction, then it was 'most likely a late deceleration'. Visser emphasized that in fetal growth retardation both 'late' and 'prolonged variable' decelerations are associated with fetal hypoxaemia at cordocentesis (Visser et al., 1990). Small variable decelerations may precede these, most probably due to decreased amniotic fluid volume and cord compression.

Neurological Morbidity

Mandruzzato enquired as to the provenance of the cases whose outcome had been studied longitudinally in terms of neurological outcome. Visser replied that they were all from the local population in Groningen, in the mid-1970s; none had been referred from outside. Neurologically morbidity was restricted to *very small* fetuses with intrauterine growth retardation, with abnormal FHR patterns, and delivered early.

Hackett et al. (1987) had reported that absence of end-diastolic flow was an especially sinister sign, associated with a high incidence of neonatal morbidity; they concluded that fetuses should be delivered before these severe waveform abnormalities occur. However, Visser noted that in this study the selected sample of fetuses were more growth-retarded and delivered at an earlier age than the 'control' fetuses with less severe waveform abnormalities. This suggests that absence of end-diastolic flow is more a marker of early and severe growth retardation—which by itself has an effect on outcome—than a marker purely related to outcome. Delivery at an earlier gestational age might lead to an even higher neonatal morbidity rate.

Visser added that the data of the 'Groningen perinatal project' were in fact identical to those of Hackett et al. (1987). Neonatal neurological morbidity was restricted to growth-retarded fetuses with antenatal heart rate decelerations; these fetuses were, however, more growth-retarded and delivered earlier, than 'control' growth-retarded fetuses that did not show antenatal decelerations (Visser, 1988). Decelerations may be considered as a sign of chronic malnutrition (including hypoxaemia) and, therefore, of severe impairment of materno-fetal exchange.

Redman then made the point that umbilical cord flow velocity measurements represented a single attribute of the fetus, related to the placental circulation, while analysis of the heart rate was a global measure, since it was modulated by many physiological variables, incorporating a measure of lower central nervous function. He asked whether a follow-up of deliveries in the late 1980s would be likely to obtain the same poor results as in the 1970s. Visser was afraid that this might be so, but agreed that terminal patterns in the FHR were now encountered less frequently. Because of better diagnostic methods the fetuses were delivered earlier and in better condition. He thought that damage in utero, before delivery, might result from chronic malnutrition; that was a hypothesis for future investigation.

Pardi pointed out that it is confusing to present data related to fetal oxygenation in terms of 'delta pO_2'. The reader does not know the original pO_2. It is true that p_aO_2 falls progressively with gestation from 20 weeks onwards. However, this is compensated by a rise in blood haemoglobin concentration, so that blood O_2 content remains fairly stable. When fetal oxygenation is expressed in terms of O_2 content, data from different groups can be compared. Visser agreed but said that such data on O_2 content were not available. In the cordocentesis data which he presented, p_aO_2 values were corrected for the duration of pregnancy, and hypoxaemia was defined as a p_aO_2 more than 2 SD below the mean for the appropriate gestational age.

Pardi said that vaginal delivery was usually associated with decreased fetal arterial pH and reduced oxygenation. Indeed the fetal pH and O_2 content fell somewhat even on caesarean section, comparing data from umbilical venous blood sampled immediately before (cordocentesis) and at caesarean section (double clampled cord). So he would not use vaginal delivery of such compromised infants. Twenty-four hours or more of regular uterine contractions could be damaging if the cervix was not ripe. Visser said that practice in the Netherlands was conservative in two senses. The caesarean rate was low (6.5%). With a normal FHR pattern, even if sometimes the umbilical flow velocity waveform was not quite normal, vaginal delivery was almost always satisfactory in growth-retarded fetuses. Antenatal management also was conservative and the induction rate was low. But they were careful, and performed elective section under general anaesthesia before the onset of labour where necessary (i.e. with antenatal signs of hypoxaemia). Redman added that, although it was primarily a concern for hospital administrators, it was cheaper to treat a fetus in utero than in neonatal intensive care, avoiding the hazards of complications such as respiratory distress and necrotizing enterocolitis before 32 weeks gestation.

General Discussion on the Diagnosis of Fetuses at Risk

In reply to questions about metabolic markers of fetal adaptation, such as rises in plasma or amniotic fluid erythropoietin, Visser agreed that with non-invasive methods exact identification of fetal health was difficult. There was not enough evidence of how quickly death occurred in utero, and the sequence of events varied with the individual; he feared invasive measures, such as cordocentesis, especially in growth-retarded fetuses early in gestation when the umbilical cord vessels were so thin. Other measures were discussed, such as NMR spectroscopy, the difficulty or impossibility as yet of measuring fetal blood pressure, and hormonal evidence of fetal adaptation (including catecholamines, ACTH and corticosteroids). It was difficult to recognize damaged fetuses; if neurological examination at birth was imprecise, what chance was there of detecting damage in utero by such means? Visser said that the Groningen data showed that 80% of neurologically abnormal infants were delivered with normal blood gas values (Huisjes et al., 1980). He quoted five papers (summarized in Visser, 1988) in which antenatal FHR abnormalities were associated with subsequent evidence of neurological morbidity. There is a major development of the brain after birth, and its plasticity might well conceal minor derangements caused by antenatal events.

The fetus certainly adapts in intrauterine growth retardation, in animals and man. There is progressive compensation for placental insufficiency and a falling p_aO_2, with a large rise in haemoglobin concentration and an increase in blood flow to the heart and brain at the expense of other organs. In animals, umbilical flow is maintained, in part by a rise in arterial pressure; we do not know if this occurs in man. Yet these adaptations are all characteristic of the mature fetus. The point was made repeatedly that we do not yet know the capacity of the early human fetus to adapt. Perhaps, Pardi suggested, in some instances adaptation may conceal the signs by which the clinician recognizes the fetus as abnormal.

References

Arduini D, Rizzo G et al. (1988) Am J Obstet Gynecol 159: 1277–1282.
Blanco CE, Martin CB, Rankin JHG et al. (1988) J Dev Physiol 10: 53–62.
Hackett GA, Nicolaides KH, Campbell S (1987) Br Med J 294: 13–16.
Huisjes HJ, Touwen BCL, Hoekstra J et al. (1980) Eur J Gynec Repro Biol 10: 247–256.
Nicolaides KH, Bradley RJ, Soothill PW et al. (1987) Lancet i: 942.
Teitel DF (1988) Sem Perinatol 12: 96–103.
Visser GHA (1988) Abnormal antepartum fetal heart rate patterns and subsequent handicap. Baillière's Clin Obstet Gynaecol 2: 117–124.
Visser GHA, Sadovsky G, Nicolaides KH (1990) Am J Obstet Gynecol 162: 698–703.
Yu YYH, Loke HL, Bajuk B et al. (1986) Br Med J 293: 1200–1203.

8

Immunological Autonomy of the Fetus

C. W. G. REDMAN

Nuffield Department of Obstetrics and Gynaecology,
John Radcliffe Hospital, Oxford, UK

The placenta and membranes form the frontier behind which the fetus can sustain its autonomy; where maternal and fetal tissues must not only coexist but establish and maintain the interchange upon which fetal survival depends. The frontier is formed during implantation and placentation, and presents the long-recognized but unresolved immunological paradox of the 'fetal allograft' (Medawar, 1954). How does the pregnant mother contrive to nourish within herself a fetus that is an antigenically foreign body?

The immune system is able to tolerate 'self' and reject 'non-self'. How this discrimination is achieved is not understood. Tolerance appears to involve three mechanisms: clonal deletion of self-reactive T-cells during thymic education early in ontogeny; clonal anergy—whereby self-reactive immune cells, usually B-cells rather than T-cells, exist but are rendered intrinsically unresponsive; and immunoregulation—the active suppression of aggressive or destructive reactions towards self antigens. In the last case a null response is achieved in the classical physiological way, by a balance between two opposing forces. It is not understood how the maternal immune system adapts to tolerate the intrauterine growth of the antigenically foreign fetus. Medawar discussed three possibilities. The anatomical separation of the mother and fetus, an absolute prerequisite for fetal autonomy, ensures that the maternal immune system is exposed only to a limited number of fetal antigens primarily confined to one specialized tissue—trophoblast. The immunogenicity of trophoblast then becomes crucial. There is clear evidence that only certain antigens are expressed, which would be expected to limit the range and magnitude of maternal immune reactions; this corresponds to the 'antigenic immaturity of the fetus'—the second of

Fetal Autonomy and Adaptation. Edited by G. S. Dawes, A. Zacutti, F. Borruto and A. Zacutti, Jr
©1990 John Wiley & Sons Ltd

Medawar's possibilities. The third, maternal immunological inertness, would in terms of today's concepts be considered to be immune tolerance, involving one of the three mechanisms already mentioned.

The Heterogeneity of Trophoblast

Trophoblast cells are heterogeneous, formed from subsets with different phenotypes found in different positions (Bulmer and Johnson, 1985). The two main classes—syncytiotrophoblast and cytotrophoblast—differentiate from trophectoderm, with which the maternal decidua first comes into contact 6 to 9 days after ovulation. Then the cytotrophoblast shell forms, after which both cytotrophoblast and syncytial elements mingle with maternal tissues. The cytotrophoblast cells are invasive at this stage, infiltrating the decidua and later the myometrium, a process which continues until at least 18 weeks (Pijnenborg et al., 1981). They also invade the decidual spiral arteries as far as the myometrial segments. In both positions—interstitial and endovascular—cytotrophoblast cells are abundant in the first half of pregnancy but have regressed almost completely by full-term.

Two areas of contact between mother and fetus are established: a large surface area, within the body of the placenta, formed by the microvillous membrane of the syncytiotrophoblast, bathed by maternal blood in the intervillous space; and a less well-defined juxtaposition of extravillous trophoblast with maternal decidual tissues. The latter includes the membranous chorion and the interstitial and endovascular cytotrophoblast in the placental bed.

Trophoblast does not invade the uterine veins in the same way as it infiltrates the arteries. But from early in the first trimester, syncytial sprouts can be detected histologically in the myometrial and endometrial veins. These cells may embolize the lungs, a well-documented process that is thought to be normal (Douglas et al., 1959). It continues throughout pregnancy so that syncytial cells can be found in uterine vein blood at term, using flow cytometric techniques (Kozma et al., 1986). Most of the embolized cells lodge in the pulmonary capillaries, arouse no inflammatory changes and are probably cleared by proteolysis (Thomas et al., 1959). Embolization is usually restricted to syncytial cells, but under pathological circumstances it may include villi (Attwood and Park, 1961) or even fragments of decidua (Cameron and Park, 1965).

Antigens of the Major Histocompatibility Complex

The antigens of the major histocompatibility complex (MHC), located on chromosome 6, control many aspects of immune reactivity and determine strong allograft rejection reactions. The genes code for two groups of cell-surface glycoproteins—class I and class II—of which some are highly polymorphic (Bodmer and Bodmer, 1985). HLA-A, -B, -C are class I MHC antigens. In the mouse, more class I genes than proteins have been defined (Goodenow et al., 1982). Apart from pseudogenes that are not expressed they include genes for differentiation antigens on lymphocyte subsets or haemopoietic tissues (Qa), and on thymocytes (Tla). Human equivalents are presumed to exist; these may include three new human class I genes that have been recently identified and designated HLA-E, -F and -G (Koller et al., 1989).

The second group, or class II MHC antigens (HLA-DP, -DQ, -DR), have a restricted tissue distribution, and are usually found only on immune cells such as lymphocytes, macrophages, and dendritic cells. T-cells recognize antigens after they have been processed by antigen-presenting cells (APC), such as macrophages. A small fragment of the processed peptide is expressed on the surface of the APC, bound to an MHC molecule, which in effect acts as an antigen receptor. The probable binding site of the class I MHC proteins—called Bjorkman's groove—has been identified (Bjorkman et al., 1987) and the physical association of class I molecules with immunogenic peptides has been demonstrated (Bouillot et al., 1989). Class II proteins probably have a similar antigen-binding function and structure.

The T-cell receptor recognizes both the antigenic peptide and the MHC molecule to which it is attached. The properties of both confer the specificity of the T-cell reaction. An antigen-specific T-cell clone will react to the antigen only when it is combined with autologous (or self) MHC proteins—the same antigen on different cells is not recognized. This is a basic immune mechanism called 'MHC restriction' (Zinkernagel and Doherty, 1979).

Engraftment creates the special case of alloreactivity in which the antigens appear to be the foreign MHC molecules themselves. Alloreactivity is characterized by its unusual strength and by the lack of MHC restriction. But there is evidence that it depends on similar mechanisms to those just described. The antigen-binding sites of MHC molecules are probably always occupied, usually not by peptides derived from foreign antigens, but by endogenous (or self) peptides; to these the organism is unresponsive because of clonal deletion or other processes of tolerance. Alloreactivity is a response not only to the foreign MHC antigen but to the many self-peptides which it normally binds. Reactivity is lost if the alloantigen is present but the character of the 'self-peptides' is changed, for example if the MHC gene is transfected into cells from another species (Heath et al., 1989).

A T-cell response is triggered by T-helper lymphocytes, which recognize then proliferate in response to antigen presented in association with class II MHC molecules (McDonald, 1982) or foreign class II proteins themselves. The helper cells stimulate the generation of cytotoxic T-cells—thought to participate in the processes of allograft rejection. However, cytotoxic T-cells are usually specific for foreign class I MHC antigens (HLA-A, -B, -C). Targets for the cytotoxic

T-lymphocytes can also be autologous cells infected with viruses, or tumour cells; in this case the specificity is 'restricted' by class I MHC products.

Thus HLA-A, -B, -C and HLA-D antigens have key roles in the generation and regulation of human T-cell-mediated immune responses, including those involved in the rejection of foreign tissues. Their expression in the placenta, particularly on the trophoblast, must be relevant to survival of the fetal allograft. HLA-D would be important as potential triggers for T-cell responses. HLA-A and -B would provide the targets for cytotoxic effector cells.

Class I Transplantation Antigens and Trophoblast

It is not known whether MHC antigens are expressed on the human morula and blastocyst although they are not expressed on cells of the early mouse embryo. In the human, neither the syncytiotrophoblast nor the underlying villous cytotrophoblast express class I MHC antigens (Faulk and Temple, 1976; Goodfellow et al., 1976; Sunderland et al., 1981) or genes (Hunt et al., 1988). In contrast, class I MHC antigens are present on many forms of non-villous trophoblast throughout gestation, including the invasive trophoblast that establishes placentation and comes into direct contact with maternal decidua and myometrium (Sunderland et al., 1981b; Redman et al., 1984, Hsi et al., 1984; Wells et al., 1984).

The class I MHC protein on trophoblast is not HLA-A, -B, or -C. It is a unique, non-polymorphic glycoprotein associated with beta-2 microglobulin, with a lower molecular weight (Ellis et al., 1986). It appears to be monomorphic so it is unlikely to function as a transplantation antigen. It has now been identified as HLA-G (Ellis et al., 1990), a product of one of a number of recently identified HLA genes of unknown function (Geraghty et al., 1987; Koller et al., 1989). At the time of writing HLA-G is not known to be expressed on human tissues other than trophoblast.

Because HLA-A, -B, -C are not expressed on trophoblast, HLA incompatibility between mother and fetus cannot be directly relevant to maternal immune recognition of trophoblast. Nor can maternal cytotoxic T-cell responses that are HLA dependent be directed towards trophoblast.

Class II Transplantation Antigens and Trophoblast

The expression of class II MHC products in the placenta is of particular interest because these are major stimuli of the rejection of allografts. HLA-DR has not been found on human syncytiotrophoblast at term (Galbraith et al., 1981) or on immature villous trophoblast, trophoblast cell columns, or the cytotrophoblast of the amniochorion (Sunderland et al., 1981). Similarly class II

MHC antigens are not expressed on murine trophoblast (Chatterjee-Hasrouni and Lala, 1979; Jenkinson and Searle, 1979).

An antibody that binds to HLA-DP, labels trophoblast from the term amniochorion and first trimester chorionic villi. However, the same cells do not bind other antibodies that react with epitopes common to all HLA-D molecules including HLA-DP. This suggests that the relevant protein is either an incomplete part of HLA-DP—for example the alpha chain on its own—or a cross-reactive but otherwise unrelated molecule (Starkey, 1987).

HLA-D-positive cells, other than trophoblast, are found in the placental villous stroma and in the connective tissue underlying the amniotic epithelium in the second and third trimester, but are never found in direct contact with maternal tissue or blood (Sutton et al., 1983). These cells have been identified as macrophages (Bulmer and Johnson, 1984; Sutton et al., 1986).

Other Antigens on Trophoblast

The absence of polymorphic histocompatibility antigens on trophoblast should make trophoblast an allogenically neutral tissue and must be the most important way in which it avoids maternal immune rejection.

But immune rejection does not depend solely on the major histocompatibility antigens. Numerous minor histocompatibility antigens can provoke rejection, although more slowly and weakly. Particular attention has been given to antigens shared by trophoblast and lymphocytes (trophoblast/lymphocyte cross-reactive antigens—TLX) (Johnson et al., 1981; Kajino et al., 1987; McIntyre, 1988), because they might modulate maternal lymphocyte function directly or indirectly. One biochemically heterogeneous TLX molecule that binds the monoclonal antibody H316 (Stern et al., 1986) has now been identified as the relatively ubiquitous membrane cofactor protein, CD46, which interacts with components of the complement system and serves to protect autologous cells from the effects of complement-mediated damage (Purcell et al., 1989). Doubtless there are other proteins, yet to be identified, that are genetically polymorphic which could lead to minor incompatibilities between mother and fetus. Placental alkaline phosphatase is probably the best characterized, being the human enzyme with the most allelic variants (Harris, 1982). But it is not known whether these trophoblast proteins lead to significant immune interactions between mother and fetus likely to influence fetal health or autonomy.

Immune Cells in the Human Decidua

The decidua is the tissue where immune recognition of trophoblast is most likely to occur. It is relevant that in the first trimester it is primarily an immune tissue, being formed mainly from cells of bone marrow origin (Bulmer and Johnson, 1984; Bulmer and Sunderland, 1984). They include macrophages, classical T-cells and large granular lymphocytes (LGLs) (Ritson and Bulmer, 1987; Starkey et al., 1988), the last being neither T- nor B-cells but sharing features with both lymphocytes and monocytes (Horwitz and Bakke, 1984). They include natural killer (NK) cells and cytolytic cells, which kill targets when they are coated with antibody. The latter population could be important if there were specific anti-trophoblast antibodies. However, the former (NK cells) attack their targets without pre-immunization, and independently of antibodies, complement, or phagocytosis. They are thought to be active in the elimination of tumour cells, can lyse cells that lack the class I MHC antigen targets needed by cytolytic T-cells (Stern et al., 1980) and have been implicated in graft rejection reactions (Gregory and Atkinson, 1984). It is also relevant that immunosuppressive activity has been ascribed to these cells (Abruzzo and Rowley, 1983). Decidual large granular lymphocytes have natural killer activity (King et al., 1989a; Ferry et al., 1990). This is a non-adaptive immune response but one which could be highly relevant if trophoblast were a target; excess activity could then be a cause of failed pregnancy, or alternatively cytolysis of trophoblast could be a mechanism for controlling the extent of implantation and placentation. But trophoblast seems to resist NK activity both in the mouse and human (King et al., 1989a; Ferry et al., 1990). NK activity can be enhanced by the action of interleukin-2; but this does not modify the reactivity against trophoblast (Ferry et al., 1990). Therefore natural killer activity seems to be irrelevant for trophoblast as far as the situation is understood.

Decidual granular lymphocytes have an unusual phenotype compared to peripheral blood LGL. They are present in the endometrium throughout the menstrual cycle but their numbers increase during the mid-secretory phase suggesting that they are under hormonal control (King et al., 1989b). It is tempting to speculate that their immune functions, which are as yet unknown, are important for the survival of the fetal allograft.

The second most common decidual immune cells are macrophages (Starkey et al., 1988). Their functions are not well investigated but they can present antigen (Dorman and Searle, 1988). If T-helper cells were stimulated by trophoblast antigens, processed by decidual macrophages, they could drive B-cells to produce specific antibodies to trophoblast. This could be one mechanism whereby specific immune responses to trophoblast could be generated. T-cells are present in the decidua—the third most common decidual immune cell—comprising about 10% of all the decidual stromal cells. When activated, T-cells express the receptor for their major growth factor, interleukin-2, but the decidual T-cells appear quiescent by this criterion (Bulmer and Johnson, 1986).

Maternal Immune Sensitization to Trophoblast

Because none of the forms of trophoblast carry class II MHC antigens they cannot stimulate maternal T-helper cells directly to trigger immune rejection. Furthermore, without expressing class I or class II MHC antigens, the villous synctiotrophoblast cannot be the target for MHC-directed cytotoxic T-cells; classical cell-mediated alloimmune responses must be irrelevant for their survival. Thus their specialized antigenic structure serves to protect this type of trophoblast. However, the extravillous trophoblast, which bears HLA-G, might be susceptible to T-cell effector function but only if the antigen were polymorphic, which so far it appears not to be. In addition, trophoblast secretes, or carries on its membrane, substances which depress lymphocyte proliferation (McIntyre and Faulk, 1979; Degenne et al., 1986); since proliferation is essential to expand the relevant clones of antigen-reactive cells this would mitigate against sensitization.

It is probable but not certain that maternal antibodies are produced against trophoblast during normal pregnancy. The Fc receptors on trophoblast, which bind free IgG non-specifically, render the detection of specific antitrophoblast antibodies difficult. But maternal antibodies (IgG and to a lesser extent IgM) to trophoblast have been reported in pregnancy sera, detected by an ELISA technique (Davies, 1985a, 1985b; Kajino et al., 1988). This finding has not yet been generally accepted and the consensus is that a specific maternal immune response to trophoblast has yet to be identified. If it is, it is not clear whether it will be important to trophoblast survival, hence placental survival and fetal autonomy.

In summary, it is not certain that the maternal immune system reacts with trophoblast. T-cell effector function, which is critical to allograft survival, is certainly irrelevant to the villous (but not necessarily the extravillous) trophoblast, whereas large granular lymphocytes could be more important. They are numerous in the decidua, in close apposition to the interstitial trophoblast, but their functions in this position are completely unknown. B-cell function should also be considered, particularly as the decidua appears to be equipped to process and present antigen.

Disorders which may Arise from Maternal Immune Reactivity to the Fetus

Two disorders of pregnancy have been proposed as being consequences of inappropriate maternal immune recognition of pregnancy—recurrent abortion (Gill, 1983; Adinolfi, 1986; Clark et al., 1987) and pre-eclampsia (reviewed by Redman and Sargent, 1986). It is speculated that trophoblast is recognized as a foreign tissue and that maternal immune rejection occurs. In the former case rejection is complete; in the latter it is incomplete—the growth and health of the placenta is compromised but pregnancy continues with later problems caused by the placental deficiencies. There is no direct evidence for these suppositions, but the first pregnancy preponderance (MacGillivray, 1958) and apparent partner specificity (Feeney and Scott, 1980) of pre-eclampsia can be explained by this and no other mechanism.

In addition there is a group of fetal disorders arising from a breakdown of the placental barrier. Feto-maternal haemorrhage sensitizes the maternal immune system to fetal antigens not expressed on trophoblast. This would be of no account if the effector arm of the maternal immune response were confined to the maternal compartment. In the case of HLA immunization, which can generate fetal-specific antibodies and cytotoxic T-cells, the maternal antibodies are absorbed harmlessly in the placenta and never reach the fetus (the placental sponge—Innes et al., 1988); the cytotoxic cells also do not normally enter the fetal compartment, or are destroyed quickly if they do (Sargent et al., 1987). In rare cases they can survive, particularly when there is an unusual degree of fetal-maternal HLA compatibility; then maternal T-cells can engraft the fetus and cause graft-versus-host disease (Pollack et al., 1982). Rhesus disease and related disorders caused by maternal-fetal blood group incompatibilities arise because maternal antibodies are actively transported to the fetus during the third trimester and are not absorbed as they cross the placenta (Rote, 1982). In the same way the fetus can passively acquire maternal autoimmune disease.

Conclusions

Medawar suggested three ways whereby the fetus could evade immune rejection by its mother. Undoubtedly anatomical separation is the most important. It is achieved by trophoblast—which, although not 'antigenically immature' is certainly specialized to restrict the extent to which it might be recognized as antigenically foreign. The mother is definitely not immunologically inert but her tolerance of trophoblast remains an enigma. Whether or not she can respond immunologically to this tissue is still in doubt. Which components of the immune system might be involved remain undefined. The maternal tissue that hosts trophoblast—the decidua—is rich in immune cells whose functions are as yet unknown. Whether recurrent abortions or pre-eclampsia can result from maternal immune intolerance of the fetus has yet to be proved. Other disturbances of fetal autonomy can arise because the placenta sometimes fails as an immune barrier.

References

Abruzzo LV and Rowley DA (1983) Homeostasis of the antibody response: immunoregulation by NK cells. Science 222: 581–585.

Adinolfi M (1986) Recurrent habitual abortion, HLA sharing and deliberate immunization with partner's cells: a controversial topic. Hum Reprod 1: 45–48.

Attwood HD and Park WW (1961) Embolism to the lungs by trophoblast. J Obstet Gynaecol Br Commonw 68: 611–617.

Bjorkman PJ, Saper MA, Samraoui B, Bennett WS, Strominger JL, Wiley DC (1987) The foreign antigen binding site and T cell recognition regions of class I histocompatibility antigens. Nature 329: 512–518.

Bodmer J and Bodmer W (1985) Histocompatibility 1984. Immunology Today 5: 251–254.

Bouillot M, Choppin J, Cornille F, Martinon F, Papo T, Gomard E, Fournie-Zaluskie M-C, Levy J-P (1989) Physical association between MHC class I molecules and immunogenic peptides. Nature 339: 473–475.

Bulmer JN and Johnson PM (1984) Macrophage populations in the human placenta and amniochorion. Clin Exp Immunol 57: 393–403.

Bulmer JN and Johnson PM (1985) Antigen expression by trophoblast populations in the human placenta and their possible immunobiological relevance. Placenta 6: 127–140.

Bulmer JN and Johnson PM (1986) The T-lymphocyte population in first trimester human decidua does not express the interleukin-2 receptor. Immunology 58: 685–687.

Bulmer JN and Sunderland CA (1984) Immunohistological characterisation of lymphoid cell populations in the early human placental bed. Immunology 52: 349–357.

Cameron HM and Park WW (1965) Decidual tissue within the lung. J Obstet Gynaecol Br Commonw 72: 748–754.

Chatterjee-Hasrouni S and Lala PK (1979) Localisation of H-2 antigens on mouse trophoblast cells. J Exp Med 149: 1238–1253.

Clark DA, Croy BA, Wegmann TG, Chaouat G (1987) Immunological and para-immunological mechanisms in spontaneous abortion: recent insights and future directions. J Reprod Immunol 12: 1–12.

Davies M (1985a) An ELISA for the detection of maternal anti-trophoblast antibodies in human pregnancy. J Immunol Methods 77: 109–118.

Davies M (1985b) Antigenic analysis of immune complexes formed in normal human pregnancy. Clin Exp Immunol 61: 406–415.

Degenne D, Canepa S, Horowitz R, Khalfoun B. Gutman N, Bardos P (1986) Effect of human syncytiotrophoblast extract on in vitro proliferative responses. Am J Reprod Immunol 8: 20–26.

Dorman PJ and Searle RF (1988) Alloantigen presenting capacity of human decidual tissue. J Reprod Immunol 191: 101–112.

Douglas GW, Thomas L, Carr M, Cullen M, Morris R (1959) Trophoblast in the circulating blood during pregnancy. Am J Obstet Gynecol 78: 960–973.

Ellis SA, Sargent IL, Redman CWG, McMichael AJ (1986) Evidence for a novel HLA antigen on human extra-villous trophoblast and a choriocarcinoma cell line. Immunology 59: 595–603.

Ellis SA, Palmer MS, McMichael AJ (1990) Human trophoblast and the chorio-carcinoma cell line BeWo express a truncated HLA class I molecule. J Immunol 144: 731–735.

Faulk WP and Temple A (1976) Distribution of beta-2 microglobulin and HLA in chorionic villi of human placentae. Nature 262: 799–802.

Feeney JG and Scott JS (1980) Pre-eclampsia and changed paternity. Eur J Obstet Gynecol Reprod Biol 11: 35–38.

Ferry B, Starkey PM, Sargent IL, Watt GO, Jackson M, Redman CWG (1990) Cell populations in the human early pregnancy decidua: natural killer activity and response to interleukin-2 of NKH-positive large granular lymphocytes. Immunology (in press).

Galbraith RM, Kantor RRS, Ferrara GB, Ades EW, Galbraith GMP (1981) Differential anatomical expression of transplantation antigens within the normal human placental chorionic villus. Am J Reprod Immunol 1: 331–335.

Geraghty DE, Koller BH, Orr HT (1987) A human major histocompatibility complex class I gene that encodes a protein with a shortened cytoplasmic segment. Proc Natl Acad Sci USA 84: 9145–9149.

Gill TJ (1983) Immunogenetics of spontaneous abortion in humans. Transplantation 35: 1–6.

Goodenow RS, McMillan M, Nicolson M, Sher BT, Eakle K, Davidson N, Hood L (1982) Identification of the class I genes of the mouse major histocompatibility complex by DNA-mediated gene transfer. Nature 300: 231–237.

Goodfellow PN, Barnstable CJ, Bodmer WF, Snary D, Crumpton MJ (1976) Expression of HLA system antigens on placenta. Transplantation 22: 595–603.

Gregory CD and Atkinson ME (1984) Large granular lymphocytes: early non-specific effector cells in allograft rejection in the mouse. Immunology 53: 257–265.

Harris H (1982) Multilocus enzyme systems and the evolution of gene expression: the alkaline phosphatases as a model example. Harvey Lect 76: 95–124.

Heath WR, Hurd ME, Carbone FR, Sherman LA (1989) Peptide-dependent recognition of H-2K(b) by alloreactive T lymphocytes. Nature 341: 749–752.

Horwitz DA and Bakke AC (1984) An Fc receptor-bearing third population of human mononuclear cells with cytotoxic and regulatory function. Immunology Today 5: 148–153.

Hsi B-L, Yeh C-JG, Faulk WP (1984) Class I antigens of the major histocompatibility complex on cytotrophoblast of human chorion laeve. Immunology 52: 621–629.

Hunt JS, Fishback JL, Andrews GK, Wood GW (1988) Expression of class I HLA genes by trophoblast cells. Analysis by in situ hybridization. J Immunol 140: 1293–1299.

Innes A, Stewart GM, Thomson MAR, Cunningham C, Catto GRD (1988) Human placenta—an antibody sponge? Am J Reprod Immunol 17: 57–60.

Jenkinson EJ and Searle RF (1979) Ia antigen expression on the developing mouse embryo and placenta. J Reprod Immunol 1: 3–10.

Johnson PM, Cheng HM, Molloy CM, Stern CMM, Slade MB (1981) Human trophoblast-specific surface antigens identified using monoclonal antibodies. Am J Reprod Immunol 1: 246–254.

Kajino T, McIntyre JA, Faulk WP (1987) Antigens of human trophoblast: trophoblast-lymphocyte cross-reactive antigens on platelets. Am J Reprod Immunol 14: 70–78.

Kajino T, McIntyre JA, Faulk WP, Cai DS, Billington WD (1988) Antibodies to trophoblast in normal pregnant and secondary aborting women. J Reprod Immunol 14: 267–282.

King A, Birkby C, Loke YW (1989a) Early human decidual cells exhibit NK activity against the K562 cell line but not against first trimester trophoblast. Cell Immunol 118: 337–344.

King A, Wellings V, Gardner L, Loke YW (1989b) Immunocytochemical characterization of the unusual large granular lymphocytes in human endometrium throughout the menstrual cycle. Human Immunol 24: 195–205.

Koller BH, Geraghty DE, DeMars R, Duvick L, Rich SS, Orr HT (1989) Chromosomal organization of the human major histocompatibility complex class I gene family. J Exp Med 169: 469–480.

Kozma R, Spring J, Johnson PM, Adinolfi M (1986) Detection of syncytiotrophoblast in maternal peripheral and uterine veins using a monoclonal antibody and flow cytometry. Hum Reprod 5: 335–336.

MacGillivray I (1958) Some observations on the incidence of pre-eclampsia. J Obstet Gynaecol Br Common 65: 536–539.

McDonald HR (1982) Differentiation of cytolytic T lymphocytes. Immunology Today 3: 183–187.

McIntyre JA (1988) In search of trophoblast-lymphocyte crossreactive (TLX) antigens. Am J Reprod Immunol 17: 100–110.

McIntyre JA and Faulk WP (1979) Trophoblast modulation of maternal allogeneic recognition. Proc Natl Acad Sci USA 76: 4029–4032.

Medawar PB (1954) Some immunological and endocrinological problems raised by the evolution of viviparity in vertebrates. Symp Soc Exp Biol 7: 320–337.

Pijnenborg R, Bland JM, Robertson WB, Dixon G, Brosens I (1981) The pattern of interstitial trophoblastic invasion of the myometrium in early human pregnancy. Placenta 2: 303–316.

Pollack MS, Kirkpatrick D, Kapoor N, Dupont B, O'Reilly RJ (1982) Identification by HLA typing of intrauterine-derived maternal T cells in four patients with severe combined immunodeficiency. New Engl J Med 307: 662–666.

Purcell DFJ, McKenzie IFC, Johnson PM, Lublin DM, Atkinson JP, Deacon NJ (1989) CD46 (HuLy-m5) antigen of humans includes the trophoblast-leukocyte antigen (TLX) and the membrane cofactor protein (MCP) of complement. Abstract P309; 4th Int Congr Reprod Immunol. J Reprod Immunol, Suppl 207.

Redman CWG and Sargent IL (1986) Immunological disorders of human pregnancy. Oxford Rev Reprod Biol 8: 223–265.

Redman CWG, McMichael AJ, Stirrat GM, Sunderland CA, Ting A (1984) Class I major histocompatibility antigens on human extra-villous trophoblast. Immunology 52: 457–468.

Ritson A and Bulmer JN (1987) Endometrial granulocytes in human decidua react with a natural-killer (NK) cell marker NKH1. Immunology 62: 329–331.

Rote NS (1982) Pathophysiology of Rh isoimmunisation. Clin Obstet Gynecol 25: 243–253.

Sargent IL, Arenas J, Redman CWG (1987) Maternal cell-mediated sensitisation to paternal HLA may occur but is not a regular event in normal human pregnancy. J Reprod Immunol 10: 111–120.

Starkey PM (1987) Reactivity of human trophoblast with an antibody to the HLA class II antigen, HLA-DP. J Reprod Immunol 11: 63–70.

Starkey PM, Sargent IL, Redman CWG (1988) Cell populations in human early pregnancy decidua: characterization and isolation of large granular lymphocytes by flow cytometry. Immunology 65: 129–134.

Stern P, Gidlund M, Orn A, Wigzell H (1980) Natural killer cells mediate lysis of embryonal carcinoma cells lacking MHC. Nature 285: 341–342.

Stern PL, Beresford N, Thompson S, Johnson PM, Webb PD, Hole N (1986) Characterization of the human trophoblast-leukocyte antigenic molecules defined by a monoclonal antibody. J Immunol 137: 1604–1609.

Sunderland CA, Naiem M, Mason DY, Redman CWG, Stirrat GM (1981a) The expression of major histocompatibility antigens by human chorionic villi. J Reprod Immunol 3: 323–331.

Sunderland CA, Redman CWG, Stirrat GM (1981b) HLA A,B,C antigens are expressed on nonvillous trophoblast of the early human placenta. J Immunol 127: 2614–2615.

Sutton L, Mason DY, Redman CWG (1983) HLA-DR positive cells in the human placenta. Immunology 49: 103–112.

Sutton L, Gadd M, Mason DY, Redman CWG (1986) Cells bearing class II MHC antigens in the human placenta. Immunology 58: 23–29.

Thomas L, Douglas GW, Carr M (1959) The continual migration of syncytial trophoblasts from the fetal placenta into the maternal circulation. Trans Assoc Am Physicians 72: 140–148.

Wells M, Hsi B-L, Faulk WP (1984) Class I antigens of the major histocompatibility complex on cytotrophoblast of the human placental basal plate. Am J Reprod Immunol 6: 167–174.

Zinkernagel RM and Doherty PC (1979) MHC-restricted cytotoxic T cells. Studies on the biological role of polymorphic major transplantation antigens during T cell restriction: specificity, function and responsiveness. Adv Immunol 27: 51–177.

Discussion

Pre-eclampsia

Thornburg asked whether there was evidence of an immunological component in pre-eclampsia; perhaps it could just be due to a malfunction of the trophoblast? Redman replied that the evidence was indirect and circumstantial. Pre-eclampsia toxaemia predominantly occurred in a first pregnancy. In subsequent pregnancies there was protection unless the partner was changed, when protection might be lost. A case-controlled study was carried out on 45 patients who, after 2–3 normal pregnancies, had developed toxaemia in a subsequent pregnancy. When the notes were reviewed the incidence of changed partnership was much greater than in the control group (Feeney and Scott, 1980). On this genetic hypothesis it was not inevitable that a change of partners would produce the right stimulus to induce toxaemia; there had to be a disorder of compatibility.

Pardi was concerned that recurrence of pre-eclampsia in a second pregnancy was as high as 35%. To this Redman replied that it was 5–10%. Some individuals had gaps in their immune repertoire, so it was not implausible that some women could not produce the response, which protected them against a second antigenic exposure. However, the immediate issue was to explain events in normal pregnancy; it would be an additional advantage if the immunological/genetic hypothesis might explain pre-eclamptic toxaemia.

Barker believed, from an ecological point of view, that the evidence pointed to a non-genetic maternal environmentally acquired causal factor in pre-eclampsia. In support of this view he cited the fact that since 1915 it had been recognized that most maternal deaths from eclampsia occurred in poorer areas, and geographically were correlated with most deaths from accidents of child birth. They were associated with poor maternal physique and health (Barker and Osmond, 1987) and were still common in the north of England and in Scotland in spite of a recent decline. This hypothesis did not preclude other factors. Redman agreed that there could well be some non-genetic influences. In populations which eat large amounts of fish-oil (containing eicosapentaenoic acid) pregnancies had longer gestational ages with heavier birthweights (Olsen et al., 1986). An effect on the incidence of pre-eclampsia had yet to be documented, but given the known effect of anti-platelet agents on the incidence of pre-eclampsia (Cunningham and Gant, 1989) and the effect of eicosapentaenoic acid on platelet function (Needleman et al., 1979) a protective effect would be expected. The level of antenatal care is another factor. When identified, pre-eclampsia can be pre-empted by a well-timed delivery. In patients who would be at death's door in two weeks, labour may be induced, and one would hardly know they had a problem. Medical intervention may be poor in poorer districts. Barker disagreed, in part because he regarded Scotland as the home of British obstetrics and because in the early years of this century many women received no antenatal care.

Animal Models

Pardi was surprised that, if Redman's hypothesis was correct, pre-eclamptic toxaemia was not present in other mammals. Redman replied that various toxaemias of pregnancy had been described in animals, though some were regarded as of biochemical origin. To study these, large breeding colonies were required, which few institutions could afford. There was a good case history of a gorilla with eclampsia, a well-documented case treated by Dr F. Zuspan, which seemed a classic instance of the human disease (Baird, 1981). In other species, with placentation similar to that of man, such as rodents, gestation was short; the issues were then different.

Local Immunity and Implantation

Patrick asked whether there were other tissues in the body which do not express transplantation immunity, like the trophoblast. Redman replied that this phenomenon was not unique to the trophoblast; it was also true of the brain and some thymus cells. The large granular lymphocytes which occur in the decidua are drawn there by some trophic influence (Croy et al., 1988). Organs successfully transplanted are not specifically surrounded by these large granular lymphocytes. When rejected the cells involved include other cell types as well. Large granular lymphocytes are not confined to the mucosal surface of the uterus; they also are present in the gut and lung.

Patrick wondered whether in view of the evidence presented, the work on recurrent abortion involving alleged suppressor factors or blocking antibodies might be premature. Redman replied that it lacked rationale. The attempt to immunize women with recurrent abortion by injection of paternal leucocytes 'to generate blocking antibodies' was no better than black magic, when it was not known what the antibodies were expected to block.

Ellendorff raised the question of whether immune recognition occurred before embryonic implantation, to which Redman replied that immune responses have a time course; they do not occur overnight. He found it difficult to believe in immunological recognition of pregnancy before implantation, although he accepted that there was biochemical recognition at an early stage.

Ellendorff also asked how the blastocyst is protected. Redman replied that no one knew the transplantation and antigenic expression of the early embryo. Though there must be a time when the early trophoblast begins to express transplantation antigens, whether this is before or after implantation no one knows. It might be possible to address this question using the methods developed for in vitro fertilization.

References

Baird J (1981) Am J Obstet Gynecol 141: 345–346.
Barker DJP and Osmond C (1987) Br Med J 295: 83–86.
Croy BA, Waterfield A, Wood W et al. (1988) Cell Immunol 115: 471–480.
Cunningham G and Gant NF (1989) New Engl J Med 321: 606–607.
Feeney JG and Scott JS (1980) Eur J Obstet Gynec Repro Biol 11: 35–38.
MacGillivray I (1958) J Obstet Gynaec Br Commonwlth 65: 536–539.
Needleman P, Raz A, Minkes MS et al. (1979) Proc Natl Acad Sci USA 76: 944–948.
Olsen SF, Hansen HS, Sorensen TIA et al. (1986) Lancet ii: 367–369.

9

Hormonal Adaption by the Fetus

J. R. G. CHALLIS, R. A. JACOBS, S. C. RILEY, K. AKAGI,
K. YANG, A. SUE-TANG, E. BERDUSCO AND A. D. BOCKING
The Lawson Research Institute, St. Joseph's Health Center, London, Ontario, Canada

It is clear that in some animals, such as sheep, maturation or activation of fetal hypothalamic-pituitary-adrenal (HPA) function, and enhanced cortisol secretion, play a pivotal role in the sequence of endocrine events leading to birth (Liggins et al., 1973; Thorburn and Challis, 1979). In addition, fetal glucocorticoids promote development and differentiation of fetal organ systems, including the lung, although they may inhibit cellular proliferation (Liggins and Kitterman, 1981; Gluckman and Liggins, 1984), and conceivably in excess could contribute to fetal growth retardation. In human pregnancy the role of the fetal adrenal in the sequence of events leading to birth is less clear (Thorburn and Challis, 1979; McNellis et al., 1987), although recent studies have suggested that cortisol may stimulate prostaglandin H_2 synthase gene expression and PGE_2 synthesis from the human fetal membranes (Potestio et al., 1988). Other effects of cortisol on organ differentiation in the human fetus are apparently similar to those described in animals (Liggins, 1977). Thus, this chapter will focus on factors concerned with maturation of the fetal HPA axis, using the sheep as an experimental model. We shall attempt to indicate deficiencies in our present knowledge, and potential areas for future investigation. Our current understanding of the mechanisms associated with activation of the HPA axis has recently been reviewed extensively, and these articles (Challis and Olson, 1988; Challis and Brooks, 1989) provide a detailed background and bibliography.

The HPA Glucocorticoid Cascade

For some time it has been accepted that there is sequential maturation of the HPA axis in fetal sheep, and that this process can be accelerated precociously

Fetal Autonomy and Adaptation. Edited by G. S. Dawes, A. Zacutti, F. Borruto and A. Zacutti, Jr
©1990 John Wiley & Sons Ltd

by administering ACTH (Liggins, 1968; Challis et al., 1982) or corticotrophin-releasing hormone (CRH) (Wintour et al., 1986; Brooks et al., 1987) to the fetus. In normal pregnancy, fetal plasma cortisol begins to rise from about day 125 (term 145–150 days), and there is now convincing evidence that this increase in cortisol is preceded by, and then continues to be associated with, a concurrent increase in the concentration of immunoreactive (IR)-ACTH in the fetal circulation (Hennessy et al., 1982; Norman et al., 1985; MacIsaac et al., 1989). These alterations in plasma ACTH and cortisol raise several questions. The progressive rise in plasma ACTH suggests either increasing hypothalamic input to the pituitary, or alterations in pituitary responsiveness to corticotrophin-releasing hormone. Further, there may be alterations in gene expression or post-translational processing of pro-opiomelanocortin (POMC). The progressive rise in total cortisol over the final 15–20 days of pregnancy occurs simultaneously with the rise in plasma ACTH. This raises questions of changes in steroid binding to plasma proteins, with changes in negative feedback, adjustments in the set point of negative feedback, as well as the possibility of additional inputs to the pituitary that overcome and/or are not subject to negative feedback controls. Recently we have proposed that cortisol itself modifies the HPA axis in a manner that reduces the efficacy of glucocorticoid negative feedback at the hypothalamic and/or pituitary level, thereby ensuring continued CRH and ACTH secretion despite elevations in fetal plasma cortisol. In addition, cortisol exerts feedforward effects on the fetal pituitary and adrenal that enhance their activation. The sheep placenta produces PGE_2 (Thorburn et al., 1988), CRH and ACTH (see below), the outputs of which, by analogy with studies in the human, may also be stimulated by cortisol and in turn provide additional trophic input to the fetal pituitary and adrenal gland. In this fashion, we suggested that a positive, feedforward cascade is established, the escape from which is birth (Challis and Brooks, 1989).

Fetal Hypothalamic Function

Both CRH and arginine vasopressin (AVP) are important hypothalamic components in the regulation of the pituitary-adrenal axis during fetal life. CRH has been measured by radioimmunoassay in extracts of medial basal hypothalamus (MBH) collected from day 100 fetuses (Brooks et al., 1989). The concentration of CRH was higher in MBH tissue collected between days 122–135, and then decreased by day 140. Brieu et al. (1989) reported a similar profile of IR-CRH change, with concentrations rising between days 123–138, but falling to day 143. In addition, these workers showed that IR-CRH was present in hypothalamic extracts obtained from fetuses at days 63–88, which is earlier than previous reports on the first appearance of CRH-containing neurones in the paraventricular nucleus at day 90 of gestation

(Levidiotis et al., 1987). These differences may relate to the lower sensitivity of immunocytochemistry than RIA. They require resolution with determination of CRH gene expression using in situ hybridization histochemistry and Northern blotting for CRH mRNA. In contrast, AVP was detected in the hypothalamus as early as days 63–88 using radioimmunoassay (Brieu et al., 1989), or by day 42 with immunocytochemistry (Levidiotis et al., 1987). Before day 132, AVP fibres terminated almost exclusively in the external lamina of the median eminence, in proximity to the primary portal capillary plexus, whereas after that time projections were made into the internal lamina of the median eminence (Levidiotis et al., 1987; MacIsaac et al., 1989). By radioimmunoassay, the ratio of IR-AVP/IR-CRH was about 5 between day 63 to day 123 of gestation, decreasing to 1.2 at term. This changing ratio may reflect the much greater efficacy of AVP as a corticotropin releasing factor in younger fetuses (Durand et al., 1987; Norman and Challis, 1987a), and the decline in potency relative to CRH with advancing gestation.

Using Sephadex G75 chromatography we were unable to find evidence for molecular weight forms of CRH larger than CRH 1–41, at least in hypothalamic extracts obtained between day 100 and term. IR-CRH was detected in human fetal hypothalami as early as 12–13 weeks gestation, and the bioactivity of this material was potentiated by addition of AVP (Ackland et al., 1986). Larger molecular weight forms of CRH, lacking biological activity, were present in hypothalami from human fetuses of 20 weeks gestational age or less, an earlier time than has been studied so far in the sheep.

Measurements of CRH mRNA are required to determine whether the decrease in hypothalamic IR-CRH concentration reflects decreased gene expression in response to elevations in plasma corticoids. In the fetal rat the levels of hypothalamic CRH mRNA increased progressively from day 17 to days 19–20, and then decreased during the perinatal period (Grino et al., 1989). In adult rats, dexamethasone micro pellets, implanted around the paraventricular nucleus (PVN), caused total inhibition of hybridizable CRH mRNA signal, whereas implants placed in other brain areas were without effect (Kovacks and Mezey, 1987). Dexamethasone also inhibited basal CRH output by fetal sheep MBH tissue perifused in vitro (Brooks et al., 1989), and since this effect was overcome by adding a depolarizing amount of potassium to the medium, the glucocorticoid effect is likely at a site other than nerve terminals. Recently, however, the significance of CRH from the PVN as a major effector of the sheep HPA axis has been questioned. In fetuses with lesions placed in the PVN, pregnancy was prolonged by 5–7 days, but birth then occurred (Gluckman PD, personal communication). Whether other sites of CRH expression, or other effectors of pituitary function are activated in these circumstances requires additional study.

The neurotransmitter regulation of CRH and AVP release in the sheep fetus has not been investigated. With the exception of serotonin, the concentration of which increases in the hypothalamus between days 130–135 and the neonatal period, most other putative neurotransmitters are unchanged (Richards et al., 1987). Exogenous metenkephalin or the analogue FK33824 stimulate increases in plasma ACTH in fetuses > 125 days of gestation, but not at days 110–115 (Brooks and Challis, 1988). This effect was blocked by the μ-receptor antagonist naloxone. Continuous administration of naloxone over 2 hours in term fetuses inhibited basal ACTH concentrations, raising the possibility of a tonic stimulatory effect of endogenous opiates on ACTH release at that time (Brooks and Challis, unpublished observations). Any opiate action is likely to be exerted at the hypothalamic rather than at the pituitary level, since specific [³H]-naloxone binding was present in hypothalamic but not pituitary membrane preparations (Yang and Challis, unpublished observations). [³H]-naloxone binding was present by day 110, suggesting that lack of opiate receptor would not account for the absence of an opiate effect on ACTH release at that time. The B_{max}, or number of specific naloxone binding sites in the hypothalamus, then increased in older fetuses (Villiger et al., 1982; Yang and Challis, unpublished observations). In the rat, opiates stimulate CRH release directly (Buckingham and Cooper, 1986), and stimulate HPA activity in part by depressing the activity of inhibitory adrenergic pathways (Buckingham and Cooper, 1987). These interactions have not been explored in fetal sheep, and may be important in relation to fetal endocrine adaptations to hypoxaemia or hypoglycaemia.

Fetal Pituitary

The fetal pituitary contains ACTH staining cells by day 40 of gestation (Perry et al., 1985) and secretes corticotrophin in vitro by day 50 (Glickman and Challis, 1980). Fragments of pro-opiomelanocortin (POMC), including pro-γ-MSH, γ-MSH, and β-endorphin/β-LPH were present in anterior pituitary cells by day 38, and in cells of the pars intermedia by day 60 of gestation (Mulvogue et al., 1986). By day 90 of pregnancy, morphologically distinct adult corticotrophs, which are angular, stellate cells that stain densely for ACTH, and fetal corticotrophs—larger, cuboidal and weakly staining cells—are distinguishable in the fetal pituitary (Perry et al., 1985; Mulvogue et al., 1986). The proportion of adult : fetal corticotrophs increases with gestational age. This altered ratio can be accelerated by intrafetal cortisol infusion, or delayed by fetal adrenalectomy (Antolovich et al., 1988). Brieu and Durand (1987) have suggested that cortisol increases the ratio of bioactive : immunological ACTH secreted by pituitary cells in vitro, and this observation correlates with the effect of cortisol in promoting appearance of the adult-type corticotroph (Antolovich et al., 1988). The mechanism of this effect, however, is unknown. It is not likely due to increased gene transcription, since the amount of total POMC mRNA, determined by slot blot analysis, decreased significantly between 100–135 days and term (days 141–144) (McMillen et al., 1988). The results of Brieu and Durand (1987) may reflect an action of cortisol on post-translational processing of POMC. Previous studies have failed to demonstrate an effect of cortisol on POMC synthesis by anterior or intermediate lobe pituitary tissue from day 120–125 fetuses, perhaps reflecting age-dependent differences in these responses (Miller and Leisti, 1984).

In vivo (Hargrave and Rose, 1986; Norman and Challis, 1987a) and in vitro (Durand et al., 1986) the fetal pituitary responds to CRH and AVP with ACTH release. AVP is more effective earlier in gestation; CRH is more effective later in fetal life, by which time the previous synergism between CRH and AVP is lost. Sustained pulsatile CRH administration in vivo enhanced the subsequent ability of pituitary cells to accumulate cAMP in response to addition of CRH in vitro (Brooks et al., 1987), but in vivo the plasma ACTH response to successive CRH pulses declined progressively during the treatment period. Long-term CRH administration did lead to premature delivery, but pituitary desensitization was again observed, and birth, in the absence of any change in the maternal peripheral plasma concentration of progesterone, could not be considered normal (Wintour et al., 1986). The possibility remains, however, that CRH may be involved in stimulating appearance of the adult (ACTH-producing) corticotroph cell type, since this effect has been observed in the rat (Gertz et al., 1987); current evidence, however, would suggest that such an effect requires the presence of cortisol. At present, it is not clear whether the fetal and adult corticotrophs are derived from a single stem cell type, or whether the former becomes (matures into) the adult cell. There is no information concerning changes in CRH or AVP responsiveness of separated fetal and adult pituitary cell types, nor on changes in the CRH or AVP receptor populations. CRH-, AVP- and CRH + AVP-stimulated ACTH release is subject to negative feedback by glucocorticoids in vivo (Wood and Rudolph, 1983; Hargrave and Rose, 1985; Norman and Challis, 1987b), and in vitro (Durand et al., 1986), but there are differences in the feedback controls of basal and stimulated ACTH release (Norman and Challis, 1987b). Basal ACTH is unaffected by exogenous glucocorticoids at days 110–115, but both basal and stimulated ACTH are decreased by exogenous glucocorticoids at >125 days (Norman and Challis, 1987b), a time after which basal ACTH and β-endorphin rise in adrenalectomized fetuses (Wintour et al., 1980). The negative feedback effect of glucocorticoids depends on the presence of glucocorticoid receptors (GR), and it has been suggested that the reduced sensitivity to cortisol-negative feedback at term (Wood, 1987) might result from a decrease in GR. Glucocorticoid receptors have been measured in cytosol (Rose et al., 1985) and in intact cells (Yang et al., 1989) from pituitaries or hypothalami of fetal sheep during pregnancy. These studies, showing substantially more GR in the pituitary than in the hypothalamus, suggest that the pituitary is the major site of glucocorticoid-negative feedback control. However, whereas pituitary GR number decreased after 4 days of intrafetal ACTH administration beginning around day 125, an effect consistent with autoregulation of GR by glucocorticoids and manifest as decreased GR gene transcription and increased GR protein clearance (Gustafsson et al., 1987), GR number rose in term pituitary tissue. Similar elevations in circulating cortisol occur at both times. The mechanism of these different effects is unknown, although current measurements of fetal pituitary GR mRNA may show whether there is any change in gene expression at term, compared to younger fetuses treated with ACTH.

Fetal Adrenal

In the human anencephalic fetus it is likely that a certain extent of fetal adrenal growth and differentiation occurs in an autonomous fashion, independent of the fetal pituitary, although influenced in part by the trophic input of placental hCG. The degree of 'autonomous' fetal adrenal growth and differentiation in fetal sheep is unknown. Whereas fetal hypophysectomy results in adrenal atrophy, the outcome on adrenal function of providing low-dose maintenance ACTH replacement to the hypophysectomized fetus has not been explored.

It is well established that there are dramatic alterations in fetal adrenal function during pregnancy. Three phases of responsiveness have been described (Madill and Bassett, 1973; Wintour et al., 1975; Glickman and Challis, 1980; Manchester and Challis, 1982). At days 50–60 the fetal adrenal secretes appreciable cortisol in response to ACTH stimulation. The responsiveness is lost in mid-gestation, but re-emerges near term. The increased responsiveness at term involves the appearance of an increased number of ACTH receptors, an increased activity of adenylate cyclase, and enhanced coupling by G_s proteins (Manchester and Challis, 1982; Saez et al., 1984). In addition, there is an increased activity of critical steroidogenic enzymes, including $P\text{-}450_{17\alpha}$ and $3\beta\text{-}HSD$ (Manchester and Challis, 1982; Saez et al., 1984). By Northern blot and in situ hybridization histochemistry it was shown that there is little mRNA in the fetal adrenal for $P\text{-}450_{scc}$, $P\text{-}450_{17\alpha}$ or $P\text{-}450_{21\beta}$ before day 49. mRNA for all three enzymes was present by day 55. However, by day 114—the period of fetal adrenal unresponsiveness—$P\text{-}450_{scc}$ and $P\text{-}450_{17\alpha}$ mRNA had decreased, whereas $P\text{-}450_{21\beta}$ was relatively unchanged. mRNAs for all three enzymes were present by day 132, and increased towards term (MacIsaac et al., 1989; Tangalakis et al., 1989). There was no relation between steroid P-450 expression and the histological distinction between 'mature' and 'immature' cells of the fetal adrenal cortex (MacIsaac et al., 1988).

Factors responsible for turning on and turning off gene expression in this model are unknown. It is interesting, however, that TGFβ (transforming growth factor β) decreases the acute stimulation of cAMP and steroid production caused by ACTH, cholera toxin or forskolin. TGFβ also inhibited the activity and amount of 17α-hydroxylase protein, and 11β- and 21-hydroxylases. Although it is a substantial step to conclude a physiological role for TGFβ, establishment of TGFβ production by adrenal cortical cells might suggest the possibility of its acting on them in a paracrine or autocrine fashion (Rainey et al., 1988).

Much attention has focused recently on the possibility that as part of the positive feedforward glucocorticoid cascade, cortisol acts on the fetal adrenal to mediate the mechanism by which ACTH activates fetal adrenal function. Liggins et al. (1977) first reported that the output of cortisol in vivo in response to an ACTH challenge was greater in fetuses that had been treated for 48 h with dexamethasone. More recently, we (Challis et al., 1985) showed that adrenal cells from fetuses pretreated in vivo with ACTH + metopirone had an attenuated capacity to accumulate cAMP or generate 11-desoxy cortisol, compared to fetuses that had received ACTH alone. The effect of metopirone on ACTH-induced maturation of these activities could be overcome by replacement cortisol. We confirmed that this effect was exerted on the capacity of cells to produce cAMP after in vitro stimulation with ACTH, rather than purely on steroidogenic enzyme activity (Challis et al., 1986; Challis and Roberts, 1988). We speculated that the likely site of cortisol mediation (action) was to increase the number or affinity of ACTH receptors (Challis and Roberts, 1988; Challis and Brooks, 1989). These results and conclusions have been confirmed by studies in adult sheep, and in adrenal cortical cells from fetuses at days 120–138 (Darbeida and Durand, 1987; Darbeida et al., 1987). Adrenal cells cultured in the presence of dexamethasone produced more corticosteroids in response to ACTH, forskolin or 8-bromo cAMP than did control cells. The effect was blocked with RU38486, the glucocorticoid receptor antagonist (Darbeida et al., 1987). Glucocorticoid pretreatment enhanced cAMP accumulation by cells treated with ACTH, but not after addition of forskolin, consistent with an effect on the ACTH receptor, as suggested above (Challis and Roberts, 1988). More recently ACTH itself has been shown to effect, in a time- and dose-dependent fashion, an increase in the number of ACTH high-affinity binding sites on bovine fasciculata cells (Penhoat et al., 1989). There was no effect on binding affinity. These studies did not examine the possibility of a mediatory role by cortisol. However, they do support the observations of an increase in ovine fetal adrenal ACTH-receptor number coincident with the increase in plasma ACTH during late pregnancy (Saez et al., 1984). The intra-adrenal effects of cortisol may be mediated by specific binding sites. The number of GR in adrenocortical cells is highest on day 100, falls to day 125, but then paradoxically increases at term, despite the possibility of auto down-regulation by high intra-adrenal and systemic cortisol concentrations at that time. Mechanisms leading to the increase in GR in term fetal adrenals are currently being examined.

Coincident with increased steroidogenic activity, there are changes in fetal adrenal growth and blood flow. Boshier and Holloway (1989) have described the decrease in total adrenocortical cell number and cell volume that occurs between day 100 and day 130, to be followed by an initial phase of hypertrophy, and then of hypertrophy and hyperplasia before term. This sequence could be explained as a primary hypertrophic response to ACTH, with ACTH then stimulating intra-adrenal IGF gene expression, which in turn stimulates hyperplasia. IGF peptides have not been localized to sheep fetal adrenals during the course of pregnancy, but are present in the fetal zone of the human fetal adrenal by immunocytochemistry (Han et al., 1987b), and their mRNAs have been localized by in situ hybridization histochemistry (Han et al., 1987a). Both ACTH and cAMP increase fetal adrenal IGF-II mRNA and this effect was partially inhibited by concurrent administration of IGF-I or IGF-II (Voutilainen and Miller, 1987, 1988). Thus, ACTH effects on adrenal growth are likely to be indirect through stimulated IGF peptides. ACTH by itself is anti-mitogenic, at least in vitro, whereas IGF-II promotes fetal adrenal cell proliferation, providing insulin is also present (Van Dijk et al., 1988). Both hyperplasia and differentiated cell responses of ovine fetal adrenal cells were promoted in vitro by IGF-I or insulin (Naaman et al., 1989). In the rat, N-terminal POMC-derived peptides (N-POMC 1–28 or N-POMC 2–28) or N-POMC 1–48/49 derived from pro-γ-MSH (N-POMC 1–74) also stimulate DNA synthesis and mitogenesis (Estivariz et al., 1988). PGE_2 has been reported to block adrenocortical mitotic activity (Szkudlinski et al., 1988). These effects have not been examined in fetal sheep adrenal tissue.

During hypoxaemia there is a 2–3-fold increase in blood flow to the fetal adrenal gland (Cohn et al., 1974), that is associated temporally with an initial rise in fetal plasma ACTH concentration (Challis et al., 1986). With time ACTH falls, but adrenal blood flow remains elevated (Challis et al., 1986). Using immunocytochemistry we have found recently that endothelial cells of the subcapsular blood vessels in the fetal adrenal contain prostaglandin H_2 synthase (PGHS) enzyme, raising the possibility that locally stimulated PG production, perhaps in response to elevated ACTH, may be responsible for changes in blood flow. At the present time, however, information is needed on blood flow distribution changes in the fetal adrenal during hypoxaemia, and the specificity of ACTH as an effector of blood flow responses needs to be examined. Other vasoactive peptides, including VIP, CRH, and perhaps endothelin, may be produced in the fetal adrenal, and elucidation of their possible roles in blood flow adaptations seems worthy of pursuit.

Placental CRH and ACTH

There is good evidence that the human placenta expresses genes for CRH and POMC, and secretes CRH and ACTH into the maternal and fetal circulation

(Robinson et al., 1988; Challis and Brooks, 1989; Jones et al., 1989). Placental CRH mRNA is similar in size to hypothalamic CRH mRNA, whereas placental POMC mRNA is 150–200 bases smaller than its pituitary counterpart (Chen et al., 1986; Frim et al., 1988). These peptides may be locally active in the placenta; for example CRH stimulates placental ACTH (Petraglia et al., 1987), and both stimulate prostaglandin output (Jones and Challis, 1989). In addition, the peptides are actively secreted into the maternal and fetal circulation (Goland et al., 1986; Campbell et al., 1987). In maternal blood, however, a high-affinity CRH-binding protein (Orth and Mount, 1987) may attenuate the biological activity of circulating CRH.

We have used immunocytochemistry to show the presence of CRH and ACTH in sheep placental tissue and fetal membranes, either in paraffin section or during monolayer tissue culture. The concentration of ACTH in these tissues rises during the second half of pregnancy, and is particularly elevated in chorion collected within 5–7 days of delivery. Evidence for placental peptide release in vivo in the sheep is limited. However, Jones et al. (1988) and we (Sue-Tang et al., unpublished observations) have shown that CRH is released dramatically into the fetal circulation in response to hypoxaemia associated with the reduction in uteroplacental blood flow. In human pregnancy, complicated by PIH, maternal plasma CRH is also elevated (Campbell et al., 1987). We have speculated that placental CRH gene transcription is increased in response to decreases in placental blood flow, hypoxaemia, or hypoglycaemia, in an attempt to maintain homeostasis through the vasodilatory effects of CRH (McCannell et al., 1982). If the compromise to the fetus is not corrected, we speculate that sustained placental output of CRH, ACTH and PGE$_2$ may augment activation of fetal HPA function, precipitating preterm labour (Challis and Hooper, 1989).

A remarkable feature of CRH regulation in women is that placental and membrane CRH mRNA and peptide output in vitro is increased by glucocorticoid treatment (Frim et al., 1988; Jones et al., 1989). Thus, a positive feedforward cascade is established in which cortisol of fetal or maternal origin, or derived from cortisone through 11-oxidoreductase activity in the amnion, stimulates CRH, which in turn stimulates placental ACTH output. These peptides are secreted into the fetal circulation to augment the drive to more cortisol secretion (Challis and Brooks, 1989). It is an intriguing possibility that a similar feedforward effect of fetal cortisol on placental CRH may apply during ovine pregnancy, and represent another facet of the prepartum glucocorticoid cascade.

CBG (Corticosteroid Binding Globulin) and Negative Feedback

Negative feedback clearly operates in the HPA axis of the ovine fetus during late pregnancy, although the sensitivity of negative feedback is reduced near term (Wood, 1987). Thus, whereas cortisol blocked nitroprusside-induced ACTH release as early as day 94 of pregnancy, the same dose of cortisol did not block nitroprusside-induced ACTH release in fetuses within 2–4 days of delivery (Rose et al., 1985; Wood, 1987). Despite the demonstration of negative feedback with exogenous cortisol, and dexamethasone, endogenous ACTH and total cortisol continue to increase over the last 25 days of gestation. However, Ballard et al. (1982) showed that the unbound corticoid concentration remained relatively stable until 1–2 days prepartum, and that late pregnancy was characterized by an increase in the fetal plasma CBG concentrations, and by a decrease in the percentage of cortisol bound to CBG. Thus, factors governing the rise in fetal CBG are important in determining the threshold for negative feedback. Ballard et al. (1983) showed that fetal CBG was not influenced by several treatments, including oestrogen or thyroid hormone administration. We found that plasma CBG was elevated during pulsatile ACTH administration to the fetus, and that this effect could be blocked with metopirone and restored with concurrent cortisol and dexamethasone treatment (Challis et al., 1985). Maternal CBG was unaltered. Thus it appeared that cortisol mediates the rise in plasma CBG, and current investigations are examining whether this results from increased CBG mRNA synthesis in fetal tissues, or from decreased CBG clearance, for example after glycosylation from the fetal circulation. Alternatively, CBG might be transferred across the placenta from the mother into the fetal compartment. This effect of cortisol in the fetus contrasts with the results from adult sheep (Berdusco and Challis, unpublished observations) and humans (Schlechte and Hamilton, 1987) where cortisol decreases the plasma CBG concentration.

The role of CBG as a plasma-binding protein is ambiguous. It seems possible that through its traditional effects of binding cortisol, negative feedback at the hypothalamus and perhaps pituitary is reduced. Alternatively, CBG may serve as a carrier protein of cortisol to other target tissues (Siiteri et al., 1982), including the placenta and membranes. There, cortisol is released after CBG binding to membrane receptor sites, or cleaved from CBG through local elastase activity. This type of mechanism might explain how CBG-cortisol interaction lowers steroid accessibility at one site, that of hypothalamo-pituitary feedback, while increasing cortisol accessibility to a second site, the placenta.

Comment

We have tried to develop the general hypothesis that in sheep activation of fetal HPA function is accompanied by several feedforward actions of cortisol, thereby effecting a maturational cascade. This concept raises several issues that require resolution, and will clearly serve as a basis for continuing investigation.

Acknowledgements

This work was supported by the Canadian Medical Research Council (Group Grants in Reproductive Biology, and in Fetal and Neonatal Health and Development), by St. Joseph's Health Center Foundation (Fellowship K. A.), by the Variety Club of Ontario (Fellowship S. C. R.), and by the Lawson Research Institute.

We thank Nan Cumming, Cheryl Lestra-Lantz, Pam Schoffer, Tami Fulford-Monahan and Doug Johnson for their help with aspects of this work, and our colleagues, especially Drs. J. E. Patrick, B. S. Richardson, V. K. Han and G. Hammond for many useful discussions.

References

Ackland JF, Ratter SJ, Bourne GL, Rees LH (1986) J Endocrinol 108: 171.
Antolovich GA, McMillen IC, Perry RA, Robinson PM, Silver M, Trahair JF, Young R (1988) In: Research in Perinatal Medicine 7: 243. Perinatology Press, Ithaca NY.
Ballard PL, Kitterman JA, Bland RD, Clyman RI, Gluckman PD, Platzker ACG, Kaplan SL, Grumback MM (1982) Endocrinology 110: 359.
Ballard PL, Klein AH, Fisher DA (1983) Endocrinology 113: 1197.
Boshier DP and Holloway H (1989) J Anat 167: 1.
Brieu V and Durand (1987) Endocrinology 120: 936.
Brieu V, Tonon M-C, Lutz-Bucher B, Durand P (1989) Neuroendocrinology 49: 164.
Brooks AN and Challis JRG (1988) J Endocrinol 119: 389.
Brooks AN, Challis JRG, Norman LJ (1987) Endocrinology 120: 2383.
Brooks AN, Challis JRG, Norman LJ (1987) Endocrinology 120: 2383.
Brooks AN, Power LA, Jones SA, Yang KP, Challis JRG (1989) J Endocrinol 122: 15.
Buckingham JC and Cooper TA (1986) Neuroendocrinology 44: 36.
Buckingham JC and Cooper TA (1987) Neuroendocrinology 46: 199.
Campbell EA, Linton EA, Wolfe CDA, Scraggs PR, Jones MT, Lowry PJ (1987) J Clin Endocrinol Metab 64: 1054.
Challis JRG and Brooks AN (1989) Endocrine Reviews 10: 182.
Challis JRG and Hooper S (1989) In: Perinatal Endocrinology, Baillière's Clinical Endocrinology and Metabolism. Saunders, New York 3: 781.
Challis JRG and Olson DM (1988) Parturition. In: The Physiology of reproduction, Vol 2 (Eds Knobil E and Neill J) p 2177, Raven Press.
Challis JRG and Roberts JM (1988) Med Sci Res 16: 353.
Challis JRG, Manchester EL, Mitchell BF, Patrick JE (1982) Biol Reprod 27: 1026.
Challis JRG, Huhtanen D, Sprague C, Mitchell BF, Lye SJ (1985) Endocrinology 116: 2267.
Challis JRG, Nancekievill EA, Lye SJ (1985) Endocrinology 116: 1139.
Challis JRG, Lye SJ, Welsh J (1986) Can J Physiol Pharmacol 64: 1085.
Challis JRG, Richardson BS, Rurak D, Wlodek ME, Patrick JE (1986) Am J Obstet Gynecol 155: 1332.
Chen C-LC, Chang C-C, Krieger DT, Bardin CW (1986) Endocrinology 118: 2382.
Cohn HE, Sacks EJ, Heymann MA, Rudolph AM (1974) Am J Obstet Gynecol 120: 817.
Darbeida H and Durand P (1987) Endocrinology 121: 1051.

Darbeida H, Naaman E, Durand P (1987) Biochem Biophys Res Commun 145: 999.

Durand P, Cathiard AM, Dacheux F, Naaman E, Saez JM (1986) Endocrinology 118: 1987.

Estivariz FE, Carino M, Lowry PJ, Jackson S (1988) J Endocrinol 116: 201.

Frim DM, Emanuel RL, Robinson BG, Smas CM, Adler GK, Majzoub JA (1988) J Clin Invest 82: 287.

Gertz BJ, Contreras LN, McComb DJ, Kovacs K, Tyrrell JB, Dallman MF (1987) Endocrinology 120: 381.

Glickman JA and Challis JRG (1980) Endocrinology 106: 1371.

Gluckman PD and Liggins GC (1984) In: Fetal Physiology and Medicine (Eds Beard RW and Nathanielsz PW), p 511.

Goland R, Wardlaw SL, Stark RI, Brown LS, Frantz AG (1986) J Clin Endocrinol Metab 63: 1199.

Grino M, Young WS, Burgunder JM (1989) Endocrinology 124: 60.

Gustafsson J, Carlstedt-Duke J, Poellinger L, Okret S, Wikstrom A-C, Bronnegard M, Gillner M, Dong Y, Fuxe K, Cintra A, Harstrand A, Agnati L (1987) Endocrine Reviews 8: 185.

Han VKM, D'Ercole AJ, Lund PK (1987a) Science 236: 193.

Han VKM, Hill DJ, Strain AJ, Towle AC, Lauder JM, Underwood LE, D'Ercole AJ (1987b) Pediatr Res 22: 245.

Hargrave BY and Rose JC (1985) Am J Physiol 249: E350.

Hargrave BY and Rose JC (1986) Am J Physiol 250: E422.

Hennessy DP, Coghlan JP, Hardy KJ, Wintour EM (1982) J Dev Physiol 4: 339.

Jones CT, Gu W, Parer JT (1988) In: Research in Perinatal Medicine 7: 107. Perinatology Press, Ithaca NY.

Jones SA and Challis JRG (1989) J Endocrinol (in press).

Jones SA, Brooks AN, Challis JRG (1989) J Clin Endocrinol Metab 68: 825.

Kovacks KJ and Mezey E (1987) Neuroendocrinology 46: 365.

Levidiotis M, Oldfield B, Wintour EM (1987) Neuroendocrinology 46: 453.

Liggins GC (1968) J Endocrinol 42: 323.

Liggins GC (1977) Am J Obstet Gynecol 126: 931.

Liggins GC and Kitterman JA (1981) In: The Fetus and Independent Life, Ciba Fdn Symposium 86.

Liggins GC, Fairclough RJ, Grieves SA, Kendall JZ, Knox BS (1973) Recent Prog Horm Res 29: 111.

Liggins GC, Fairclough RJ, Grieves SA, Forster CS, Knox BS (1977) In: The Fetus and Birth, Ciba Foundation Symposium 47, p 5. Elsevier, Amsterdam.

MacIsaac RJ, Hammond VE, Levidiotis M, Tangalakis K, Wintour EM (1988) In: The Liggins Symposium. Perinatology Press, Ithaca NY (in press).

MacIsaac RJ, Hammond VE, Levidiotis M, Tangalakis K, Wintour EM (1989) In: Advances in Fetal Physiology, p 321. Perinatology Press, Ithaca NY.

Madill D and Bassett JM (1973) J Endocrinol 58: 75.

Manchester EL and Challis JRG (1982) Endocrinology 111: 889.

McCannell KL, Lederis K, Hamilton PL, Rivier J (1982) Pharmacology 25: 116.

McMillen IC, Mercer JE, Thorburn GD (1988) J Mol Endocrinol 1: 141.

McNellis D, Challis JRG, MacDonald PC, Nathanielsz PW, Roberts JM (1987) (Eds) National Institute of Child Health & Human Development Research Planning Workshop, Nov 29–Dec 1. Perinatology Press, Ithaca NY.

Miller WL and Leisti S (1984) Endocrinology 115: 249.

Mulvogue HM, McMillen IC, Robinson PM, Perry RA (1986) J Develop Physiol 8: 355.

Naaman E, Chatelain P, Saez JM, Durand P (1989) Biol Reprod 40: 570.

Norman LJ and Challis JRG (1987a). Endocrinology 120: 1052.

Norman LJ and Challis JRG (1987). Can J Physiol Pharmacol 65: 1186.

Norman LJ, Lye SJ, Wlodek ME, Challis JRG (1985) Can J Physiol Pharmacol 63: 1398.

Orth DN and Mount CD (1987) Biochem Biophys Res Commun 143: 411.

Penhoat A, Jaillard C, Saez JM (1989) Proc Natl Acad Sci USA 86: 4978.

Perry RA, Mulvogue HM, McMillen IC, Robinson PM (1985) J Develop Physiol 7: 397.

Petraglia F, Sawchenko PE, Rivier J, Vale WW (1987) Nature 328: 717.

Potestio FA, Zakar T, Olson DM (1988) J Clin Endocrinol Metab 67: 1205.

Rainey WE, Viard I, Mason JE, Cochet C, Chambaz EM, Saez JM (1988) Mol Cell Endocrinol 60: 189.

Richards GE, Gluckman PD, Manelli SC (1987) Life Sci 41: 1881.

Robinson BG, Emanuel RL, Frim DM, Majzoub JA (1988) Proc Natl Acad Sci USA 85: 5244.

Rose JC, Hargrave BY, Dix PM, Meis PJ, LaFave M, Torpe B (1985) Am J Obstet Gynecol 151: 1128.

Rose JC, Kute TE, Winkler L (1985) Am J Physiol 249: E345.

Saez JM, Durand P, Cathiard A-M (1984) Mol Cell Endocrinol 38: 93.

Schlechte JA and Hamilton D (1987) Clin Endocrinol (Oxf) 27: 197.

Siiteri PK, Murai JT, Hammond GL, Nisker JA, Raymouve WJ, Kuhn RW (1982) Rec Prog Horm Res 38: 457.

Szkudlinski M, Lewinski A, Zerekmelen G, Sewerynek E (1988) Neuroendocrinology Letters 10: 317.

Tangalakis K, Coghlan JP, Connell J, Crawford R, Darling P, Hammond VE, Haralambidis J, Penschow J, Wintour EM (1989) Acta Endocrinologica (Copenh) 120: 225.

Thorburn GD and Challis JRG (1979) Physiol Rev 59: 863.

Thorburn GD, Hooper SB, Rice GE, Fowden AL (1988) Luteal regression and parturition. In: The Onset of Labor, p 185. Perinatology Press, Ithaca NY.

Van Dijk JP, Tanswell AK, Challis JRG (1988) J Endocrinol 119: 509.

Villiger JW, Taylor KM, Gluckman PD (1982) Pediatric Pharm 2: 349.

Voutilainen R and Miller W (1987) Proc Natl Acad Science USA 84: 1590.

Voutilainen R and Miller WL (1988) DNA 7: 9.

Wintour EM, Brown EH, Denton DA, Hardy KJ, McDougall JG, Oddie CJ, Whipp GT (1975) Acta Endocrinol (Copenh) 79: 301.

Wintour EM, Coghlan JP, Hardy KG, Henessey DP, Lingwood BE, Scoggins BA (1980) Acta Endocrinol (Copenh) 95: 546.

Wintour EM, Bell RJ, Carson RS, MacIsaac RJ, Tregear GW, Vale W, Wang X-M (1986) J Endocrinol 111: 469.

Wood CE (1987) Am J Physiol 252: R624.

Wood CE and Rudolph AM (1983) Endocrinology 112: 1930.

Yang K, Jones SA, Challis JRG (1989) Endocrinology 126: 11.

Discussion

Early Gene Expression in the Hypothalamus and Pituitary

Ellendorff asked whether CRH of central origin might be activating the fetal pituitary at an early age. Could POMC gene expression occur early in fetal life, with leakage to the pituitary and/or adrenal glands? Challis replied that POMC gene products had been identified cytochemically as early as 40 days gestation. Using immunocytochemical methods pro-γMSH, ACTH and β-endorphin had been identified in the fetal pituitary a few days before the hypothalamic-pituitary portal vascular connections were established. He speculated that in sheep CRH and POMC gene expression might be activated yet earlier in a compromised situation. In man placental CRH is more important, and there is good evidence that the glucocorticoids activate placental CRH gene expression. This initiates an intraplacental paracrine feedforward loop as: cortisol → CRH → ACTH, which leads to prostaglandin production locally.

In reply to a question from Simpson regarding temporal expression of AVP, Challis said he had referred only to immunoassay and histochemical data to show that AVP was present in the hypothalamus by day 42 of gestation. Biologically active ACTH is present in fetal pituitary cells by day 50. Pituitary cells from the fetal lamb on day 50, co-incubated with adult adrenal cells, induce cortisol secretion from the latter. Therefore, POMC expression and processing leads to ACTH secretion from the pituitary at the same time as the (early) expression of steroidogenic enzymes in the adrenal glands. The concentration of ACTH in fetal plasma at that time is not known.

Challis did not know why cortisol was produced so early in fetal lambs; there was no evidence. The fact that in sheep and cows cortisol expression was turned off in mid-gestation, after the initial release, could be interpreted as protection against the induction of premature labour.

The Onset of Parturition

Dawes asked what actually precipitated labour in sheep. Ever since Liggins' observations (Liggins, 1969) that fetal hypophysectomy prevented parturition, this had been a matter for debate. What was the initiating factor that normally determined parturition so accurately (147 ± 2 days) in this species?

In reply Challis referred to the unpublished experiments of Gluckman, who found that ablation of the paraventricular nucleus only prolonged pregnancy in sheep by 4–5 days. This was disappointing. The failure to prolong pregnancy further could be due to the availability of CRH from other sources. But Ellendorf was not surprised at the result. He pointed out that the accessory system was diffusely distributed in the hypothalamus, and could affect the pituitary. There was also the possibility of AVP release from the supraoptic nucleus, and evidence of leakage from the posterior to the anterior pituitary.

Ellendorff said that it was customary to relate the events of parturition to change in the plasma levels of hormones. But there was a large gap in time between gene expression and the detection of the end product in the plasma. More attention should be paid to local effects by diffusion or through the microcirculation. Concepts would need revision when we understood what controls gene expression and where its products go. Challis agreed wholeheartedly. That was why he had emphasized the effect of growth factors acting on the adrenal gland to control growth and vascularization in a paracrine fashion, and also the paracrine control in the placenta of the cascade involving CRH, POMC and glucocorticoids.

Challis went on to say that in man the evidence suggested a more complex control of parturition, involving not only a feedforward cascade from hypothalamus, pituitary, adrenal, and myometrium but also an important role for a local cascade involving CRH and ACTH in the placenta. Both CRH and ACTH could be released from the placenta to affect the fetal pituitary, and hence (through further ACTH release) to accelerate cortisol release from the adrenal (see Challis and Brooks, 1989). He referred to stimulation by cortisol of CRH gene expression in human placenta, which might be regarded as paradoxical since cortisol classically turns off CRH gene expression in the hypothalamus. Consequently human labour can be modulated in many other ways. Dawes raised the possibility that this might explain the more variable length of human gestation.

References

Challis JRG and Brooks AN (1989) Endocrine Reviews 10: 182–204.
Liggins GC (1969) In: Foetal Autonomy (Eds: Wolstenholme GEW and O'Connor M) Ciba Fdn Symp 10: 182–204.

10

Regulation of Genes Encoding Steroidogenic Enzymes During Fetal Development

E. R. SIMPSON, J. I. MASON, J. LUND, R. AHLGREN,
D. T. STIRLING AND M. R. WATERMAN
University of Texas Southwestern Medical Center, Dallas, Texas, USA

In ruminant species such as sheep and cattle, there is a pronounced rise in fetal plasmal levels of cortisol towards the end of gestation. This is generally perceived to be a signal for initiation of parturition and the onset of labour (Liggins et al., 1977). A number of studies have indicated that glucocorticoids cause an increase in 17α-hydroxylase expression in the placenta of such species towards term (Flint et al., 1975; France et al., 1988), and it is believed that this induction allows the synthesis of oestrogen by the placenta, which provides, in turn, a signal for initiation of parturition (Thorburn and Challis, 1979). In sheep, secretion of cortisol by the fetal adrenal appears to follow changes in the fetal plasma levels of ACTH, which also rise late in gestation (Jones et al., 1977; MacIsaac et al., 1985). The adult adrenal is under both acute and chronic control by ACTH (Waterman and Simpson, 1987). The acute response leads to a rapid mobilization of substrate cholesterol to the inner mitochondrial membrane resulting in enhanced steroidogenesis; this is mediated by cyclic AMP. The chronic effect of ACTH on the adrenal cortex includes the transcriptional activation of the genes encoding the steroid hydroxylases, namely cholesterol side-chain cleavage ($P-450_{scc}$), 17α-hydroxylase ($P-450_{17\alpha}$), 21-hydroxylase ($P-450_{C21}$) and 11β-hydroxylase ($P-450_{11\beta}$), as well as the mitochondrial iron-sulphur protein, adrenodoxin (John et al., 1986). The activation appears to be mediated by labile protein factors that are synthesized as a primary response to ACTH-mediated elevation of intracellular cyclic AMP levels. However, there is evidence that other factors may be involved in the regulation of expression

Fetal Autonomy and Adaptation. Edited by G. S. Dawes, A. Zacutti, F. Borruto and A. Zacutti, Jr
©1990 John Wiley & Sons Ltd

of these enzymes also. For example, it is known that when adult bovine adrenal cells are placed in culture in the absence of ACTH, whereas P-450$_{17\alpha}$ levels become undetectable within a few days, the levels of P-450$_{scc}$ remain detectable, indicating that perhaps some other factor is maintaining basal levels of P-450$_{scc}$, but not of P-450$_{17\alpha}$ (Zuber et al., 1985). Addition of ACTH to such cultures results in an increase in the expression of all of these enzymes.

In addition to stimulatory factors, there are other factors which are inhibitory of expression of these enzymes; for example, when the expression of P-450$_{17\alpha}$ is induced by ACTH this effect is markedly inhibited by phorbol esters as well as the growth factor TGF-β (McAllister and Hornsby, 1987; Rainey et al., 1988b). On the other hand, P-450$_{scc}$ as well as 3β-hydroxysteroid dehydrogenase levels are either unchanged or else increased to some extent by TGF-β administration. In an attempt to understand the molecular mechanisms underlying the changes in steroidogenesis which take place in the fetal adrenal, the levels of mRNA encoding the various steroidogenic enzymes in the fetal adrenal of the bovine throughout gestation have been studied, as well as the levels of enzyme protein, by Western blotting analysis (Lund et al., 1988).

Levels of Steroidogenic Proteins and Their mRNA Species Throughout Gestation in the Bovine Fetal Adrenal

When the level of P-450$_{17\alpha}$ protein was examined in fetal bovine adrenal homogenates from fetuses of various ages (Figure 1) it was observed that protein was undetectable in adrenals from fetuses of around 17 cm CVR (gestational age, GA 100 days) and remained undetectable until late in gestation, becoming detectable in adrenal protein preparations of fetuses of greater than 75 cm CVR (GA 240 days). (CVR is the length of each fetus measured from the crown along the vertebrae to the rump.) However, surprisingly, the adrenals from fetuses of younger gestational age also exhibited high levels of P-450$_{17\alpha}$ protein. Protein was first detectable in fetuses of around 7 cm CVR (GA 50 days), the levels increased and reached a maximum in fetuses of 9–10 cm CVR (GA 60–70 days) and then declined to undetectable levels. In contrast, P-450$_{scc}$, P-450$_{C21}$, P-450$_{11\beta}$, and adrenodoxin were detectable in adrenal protein preparations from fetuses throughout gestation (Figure 1). The smallest fetuses from which adrenals could be removed expressed these proteins, and whereas the levels of these proteins increased and decreased in concert with the levels of P-450$_{17\alpha}$, they remained at detectable levels throughout gestation.

To determine whether the observed differences in the levels of the various P-450 proteins were reflective of differences in the respective mRNA levels, Northern blots were performed. As shown in Figure 2, P-450$_{17\alpha}$ mRNA was clearly detectable in adrenal RNA preparations from fetuses of 6.5 to 16 cm CVR and from fetuses of 75 cm CVR and larger. On the other hand, P-450$_{17\alpha}$

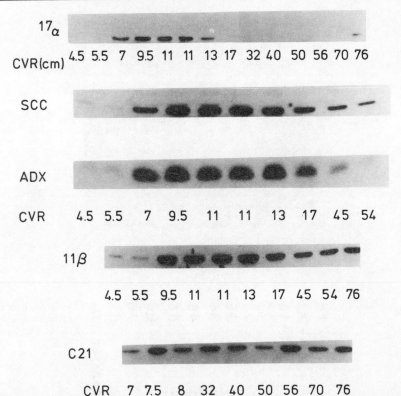

17_α

CVR(cm) 4.5 5.5 7 9.5 11 11 13 17 32 40 50 56 70 76

SCC

ADX

CVR 4.5 5.5 7 9.5 11 11 13 17 45 54

11β

4.5 5.5 9.5 11 11 13 17 45 54 76

C21

CVR 7 7.5 8 32 40 50 56 70 76

FIGURE 1 Immunoblot analysis of steroid hydroxylases in fetal bovine adrenal homogenates. Homogenates of adrenals from bovine fetuses of various gestational ages were subjected to SDS-PAGE (100 μg protein/lane), blotted to nitrocellulose and probed with monospecific antibodies. CVR (cm) is the length of each fetus as measured from the crown along the vertebrae to the rump and is related to the gestational age (20 cm ≈ 100 days, and 80 cm ≈ 280 days). 17α = 17α-hydroxylase; scc = cholesterol side-chain cleavage; ADX = adrenodoxin (a component of the cholesterol side-chain cleavage system); 11β = 11β-hydroxylase; C21 = C21-hydroxylase

mRNA was undetectable during mid-gestation. Thus the on-off-on pattern of P-450$_{17\alpha}$ protein in bovine fetal adrenals appears to be associated with the episodic presence of P-450$_{17\alpha}$ mRNA. A corresponding Northern blot of P-450$_{scc}$ mRNA showed significant levels of this RNA throughout gestation.

To determine whether fetal adrenal steroid synthesis was reflective of these changes in the levels of steroidogenic enzymes, cortisol and corticosterone levels in fetal adrenal homogenates were determined. It was observed that the levels of cortisol present in the adrenal homogenates paralleled the levels of P-450$_{17\alpha}$ mRNA and protein, in that the levels were high at early and late stages of gestation, whereas they were essentially undetectable at mid-gestation. On the other hand, corticosterone was detectable in adrenal homogenates from fetuses

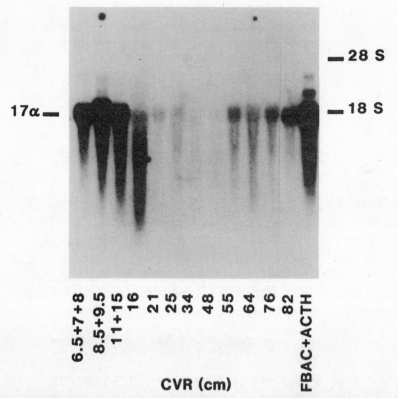

FIGURE 2   Northern blot analysis of adrenal P-450$_{17\alpha}$ (17α) RNA from bovine fetuses of various gestational ages. Total adrenal RNA (50 μg) from bovine fetuses of varying GA, as indicated by their CVR in centimetres, was size-fractionated on 1.25% agarose/formaldehyde gels and Northern blotted. The filters were hybridized with a p-450$_{17\alpha}$-specific bovine cDNA that had been ^{32}P-labelled. The positions of 18 S and 28 S RNA are marked. The lane marked FBAC + ACTH contained RNA prepared from cultured fetal bovine adrenal cells (40 cm CVR) that were treated with ACTH (0.1 μM) for 24 h

throughout gestation. This is to be expected because of the requirement for 17α-hydroxylase for cortisol production, but not that of corticosterone.

To determine the role of ACTH in this episodic pattern of fetal adrenal steroidogenesis, ACTH in bovine fetal plasma was determined throughout gestation. It was observed that the ACTH levels were high in fetuses smaller than 30 cm CVR, and in fetuses larger than 70 cm CVR, but were extremely low in the mid-gestational period. Thus, it appears that the levels of P-450$_{17\alpha}$ mRNA and protein as well as the corresponding levels of cortisol were clearly reflective of the changing levels of ACTH in the bovine fetal plasma throughout gestation. On the other hand, levels of the other steroidogenic enzymes, namely

P-450$_{scc}$, P-450$_{11\beta}$, P-450$_{C21}$, and adrenodoxin, were readily detectable at mid-gestation and clearly did not correlate with the ACTH levels at this time, suggesting once again that other factors in addition to ACTH might be involved in the regulation of these steroidogenic enzymes, in contrast to P-450$_{17\alpha}$. Further support for the importance of ACTH as a regulator of fetal adrenal P-450$_{17\alpha}$ was obtained from studies using primary cultures of fetal bovine adrenal cells obtained from fetuses at the mid-gestational period when adrenal P-450$_{17\alpha}$ was absent. Western and Northern blot analysis revealed that when cells were cultured for 3 days and then treated for 24 hours in the presence or absence of ACTH, no P-450$_{17\alpha}$ protein or mRNA was detectable in the control cells, whereas treatment with ACTH resulted in a large increase in the levels of both P-450$_{17\alpha}$ mRNA and P-450$_{17\alpha}$ protein. A similar result was obtained with dibutyryl cyclic AMP. These data further support the conclusion that it is the absence of ACTH during mid-gestation that is responsible for the absence of P-450$_{17\alpha}$ during this period; however, the cells retained the capacity to be responsive to hormone during mid-gestation. On the other hand, when the levels of P-450$_{scc}$, P-450$_{C21}$, P-450$_{11\beta}$, and adrenodoxin were determined in these cells by Western blotting, the control cells contained detectable levels of each protein, whereas the ACTH-treated cells showed increased levels, albeit not to the extent of the increase observed with P-450$_{17\alpha}$.

Similar data to these obtained with the bovine fetal adrenal have been obtained in studies using sheep fetal adrenal. In sheep where fetal ACTH levels are known to be extremely low prior to about 136 days of gestation (John et al., 1987), P-450$_{scc}$ and P-450$_{11\beta}$ are readily detectable as early as 85 days of gestation whereas P-450$_{17\alpha}$ is undetectable at that time. Furthermore, in a similar fashion to the bovine fetus, fetal adrenal steroidogenesis is expressed at high levels very early in gestation in the sheep (Tangalakis et al., 1989). The reason for this fetal adrenal activity early in gestation in the ruminant species is unclear at this time, but may reflect a requirement for cortisol for developmental processes relatively early in gestation.

Expression of Steroidogenic Enzymes in the Fetal Testis and Ovary of the Bovine

In parallel with these studies on the fetal adrenal, corresponding determinations have been conducted on fetal testis (Lund et al., 1988) and ovaries throughout gestation. P-450$_{17\alpha}$ and P-450$_{scc}$ were detectable in testis homogenates from fetuses as small as 4.5 cm CVR. The levels of the proteins increased and decreased in a temporal pattern similar to that of the adrenal. However, whereas adrenal P-450$_{17\alpha}$ was absent during mid-gestation, testicular P-450$_{17\alpha}$ remained at detectable levels throughout gestation. By contrast, in the case of the ovary, low levels of ovarian P-450$_{scc}$ but not P-450$_{17\alpha}$ could be detected in fetuses of

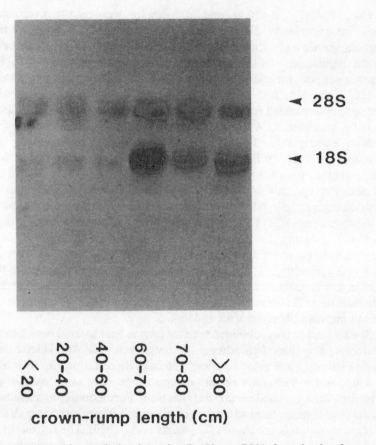

◄ 28S

◄ 18S

FIGURE 3   Northern blot analysis of ovarian P-450₁₇α mRNA from bovine fetuses of various gestational ages. Total ovarian RNA (50 μg) from bovine fetuses of varying GA, as indicated by their CVR in centimetres, was size-fractionated on 1.25% agarose/formaldehyde gels and subjected to Northern blot analysis as described in the legend to Figure 2

less than 60 cm CVR. However, in bovine fetuses of 60 cm or greater CVR a dramatic change in the microscope appearance of the ovary was evident (Stirling et al., unpublished observations). These ovaries were observed to contain follicle-like structures. Microscopy reveals that these are fluid-filled and apparently contain granulosa cells surrounding the basement membrane as well as an ovum. In addition, some of these appear to have undergone, at a later stage of gestation—greater than 70 cm CVR, a quasi-luteinization in that although the oocyte was not shed, the follicular space was nonetheless filled with blood.

Similar observations have been made in a number of other species, including sheep and human. This appearance of follicular-like structures in bovine fetuses greater than 60 cm CVR was accompanied by a dramatic increase in the levels of both $P\text{-}450_{scc}$ and $P\text{-}450_{17\alpha}$ protein and mRNA (Figure 3) (Stirling et al., unpublished observations). This expression declined somewhat but not to zero at the stage of quasi-luteinization greater than 70 cm CVR. The significance of this gestational ovarian development is unclear. At present we are attempting to relate these changes in steroidogenic enzyme expression in fetal ovary and testis to fetal plasma gonadotrophin levels as well as to those of steroids.

Steroidogenesis in the Human Fetal Adrenal

In contrast to ruminant species, steroidogenesis in the human fetal adrenal is readily apparent throughout gestation. Miller and coworkers (Voutilainen and Miller, 1987) have measured the mRNA levels for $P\text{-}450_{scc}$ and $P\text{-}450_{17\alpha}$ in human fetal adrenals within a narrow range of gestational age (14–20 weeks); no significant changes in $P\text{-}450_{scc}$ and $P\text{-}450_{17\alpha}$ mRNA levels could be detected although expression of these RNA species was readily apparent. In human fetal testis, on the other hand, $P\text{-}450_{scc}$ and $P\text{-}450_{17\alpha}$ mRNA transcripts were more abundant between 14 and 16 weeks of gestational age than between 20 and 26 weeks of gestational age, which is a time shortly after maximal levels of hCG are found in the fetal plasma. In contrast, the corresponding mRNA levels in the ovary were very low throughout this period. Studies of human fetal adrenal cells in culture have revealed that the expression of these enzymes is regulated by ACTH via cyclic AMP (DiBlasio et al., 1987) and that cyclic AMP-independent factors such as phorbol esters have differential effects on the expression of these enzymes (Mason et al., 1986) in a similar fashion to those demonstrated in adult bovine adrenal cells in culture. It appears then that in the case of the human fetal adrenal, as well as the bovine fetal adrenal, factors other than ACTH may also be important in maintaining expression of these enzymes. In this context it was observed in adrenals from anencephalic human fetuses, which are characterized by extremely low ACTH levels, that $P\text{-}450_{17\alpha}$ and $P\text{-}450_{scc}$, as well as $P\text{-}450_{11\beta}$, $P\text{-}450_{C21}$, and adrenodoxin, were all present at levels corresponding to adrenal from normal fetuses (John et al., 1987), in spite of the fact that adrenal adenylate cyclase activity was extremely low and unresponsive to ACTH (Carr, 1986). The reason for this apparent cyclic AMP-independent expression remains to be determined.

Regulation of Expression of Steroidogenic Cytochrome P-450 Species

In order to gain further insight into the regulatory mechanisms involved in expression of these enzymes, we have commenced studies designed to dissect the transcriptional regulation of the genes encoding bovine $P-450_{scc}$ and bovine $P-450_{17\alpha}$ (Ahlgren and Lund, unpublished). These studies have been conducted by preparing a series of deletion mutations of the $5'$-end of the genes encoding these two proteins. These segments of the $5'$ flanking region were then inserted into chimaeric constructs containing either the CAT reported gene or else the β-globin reporter gene. These plasmids were then used to transfect either Y-1 mouse adrenal tumour cells or else adult bovine adrenal cells in culture. On the basis of these studies, cis-acting elements with the $5'$ region of both of these genes have been identified which confer cyclic AMP responsiveness to these chimaeric constructs. In the case of the $P-450_{17\alpha}$ gene, this is found between -243 and -255 bp upstream from the start of transcription, whereas in the case of the $P-450_{scc}$ gene, this is found between -186 and -101 bp upstream from the start of transcription. In neither case was any homology found to the consensus cyclic AMP-responsive element (CRE; TGACG TCA) or to the AP-2 binding site (CCCCAGGC) within this region, indicating that the mechanisms for conferring cyclic AMP responsiveness to these steroidogenic genes are quite different from those of other genes which have so far been characterized. We are at present attempting to define other regions of these genes which confer responsiveness to cyclic AMP-independent factors, such as phorbol esters and growth factors.

Conclusions

Although studies on the regulation of expression of these steroidogenic genes are in their infancy, the long-term goal is to provide a molecular explanation for the episodic pattern of expression of these enzymes in the ruminant fetal adrenal throughout gestation. This will involve identifying regions of these genes which confer both cyclic AMP-dependent and cyclic AMP-independent responsiveness to the genes. In addition, it will require identifying the factors present in the fetal plasma which mediate the cyclic AMP- and ACTH-independent expression.

References

Carr BR (1986) J Clin Endocrinol Metab 63: 51–55.
DiBlasio AM, Voutilainen R, Jaffe RB, Miller WL (1987) J Clin Endocrinol Metab 65: 170–175.
Flint APF, Anderson ABM, Steele PA, Turnbull AC (1975) Biochem Soc Trans 3: 1189–1194.
France JT, Magness RR, Murry BA, Rosenfeld CR, Mason JI (1988) Mol Endocrinol 2: 193–199.

John ME, John MC, Boggaram V, Simpson ER, Waterman MR (1986) Proc Natl Acad Sci USA 83: 4715–4719.

John ME, Simpson ER, Carr BR, Magness RR, Rosenfeld CR, Waterman MR, Mason JI (1987) Mol Cell Endocrinol 50: 263–268.

Jones CT, Boddy K, Robinson JSJ (1977) Endocrinol 72: 293–300.

Liggins GC, Fairclough RJ, Grieves SA, Forster CS, Knox BS (1977) In: The Fetus and Birth, Ciba Fnd Symp 47: 5–25.

Lund J, Faucher DJ, Ford SP, Porter JC, Waterman MR, Mason JI (1988) J Biol Chem 263: 16195–16201.

MacIsaac RJ, Bell RJ, McDougall JG, Tregear GW, Wang X, Wintour EM (1985) J Dev Physiol 7: 329–338.

Mason JI, Carr BR, Rainey WE (1986) Endocrine Res 12: 447–467.

McAllister JM and Hornsby PJ (1987) Endocrinology 121: 1908–1910.

Rainey WE, Viard J, Mason JI, Cochet C, Chambaz EM, Saez JM (1988) Mol Cell Endocrinol 60: 189–198.

Tangalakis K, Coghlan JP, Connell J, Crawford R, Darling P, Hammond VE, Haralambidis J, Penschow J, Wintour EM (1989) Acta Endocrionol (Copenh) 120: 225–232.

Thorburn GD and Challis JRG (1979) Physiol Rev 59: 863–916.

Voutilainen R and Miller WL (1987) J Clin Endocrinol Metab 63: 1145–1150.

Waterman ER and Simpson ER (1987) Rev Biochem Toxicol 8: 259–287.

Zuber MX, Simpson ER, Hall PF, Waterman MR (1985) J Biol Chem 260: 1842–1848.

Discussion

In reply to questions from Ellendorff, Simpson agreed that the precise times over which enzymes were expressed were very important. There were two elements of uncertainty in his data. The first concerned the fact that tissues were obtained in the rough and tumble of a slaughterhouse. The age of the fetus was determined from its size, but that was also determined by nutrition and other factors. Secondly, there might be a gap between the expression of the message and the appearance of an enzyme in measurable quantities. The example of placental 17-hydroxylase (Al Conley, Dallas; unpublished observations) was relevant, since in this case mRNA encoding of this enzyme appeared several days before protein. Certainly the accuracy of measurement was rate-limiting.

Dawes asked whether anything was yet known of the clock which regulated gene expression with time. Simpson replied that he'd like to know too; we'd have to wait. Ellendorf speculated that this could perhaps be addressed by challenging the fetus with steroids or ACTH, but Simpson would prefer to do this in cell cultures rather than in whole animals. He hoped that within a short time the fetal plasma levels of hormones in mid-gestation would be known. It was still not evident to Dawes how this could answer the question.

Mechanisms of Regulation

Challis then raised the question of how enzymes such as 17-hydroxylase were specifically inhibited early in gestation. Could it be due to the action of an inhibitory growth factor such as TGFβ. Simpson replied that in a number of tissues, fetal and adult adrenal and the ovarian theca, TGFβ does inhibit 17-hydroxylase, possibly in part by an action on protein kinase C.

Challis wondered, if it were assumed that TGFβ does inhibit 17-hydroxylase expression, whether TGFβ might interfere with the production of cAMP binding protein? Or does it facilitate production of some other protein with an indirect action? There was no direct information. Simpson quoted the effect of glucocorticoids on the POMC gene as appearing to be due to binding close to the cAMP area, inducing interference therewith. That was a possible model; it was guesswork.

Choice of Animal Species

Dawes wondered whether the search for truth was facilitated by working on species such as man, where there were many ethical problems, or other large expensive mammals. Perhaps marsupials would be regulated by simpler mechanisms, so far as paturition was concerned. In problems of genetic regulation the fruit fly and the earthworm were said to show particular advantages.

Ellendorf quoted work on the olfactory system of marsupials (Ellendorff et al., 1988) that proved they were very suitable animal species in which to study developmental physiology. In many species studies on the development of the special senses were difficult. In young wallabies (*Macropus eugenii*) the central components of the visual system were laid down after birth when the joey was more accessible. He had found the chicken embryo useful as an alternative. Simpson was sure that the critical issue was to ask the right question. The development of the nematode, *C. elegans*, had been studied so thoroughly that the life history of every cell had been traced.

Challis then asked Redman whether there were species, other than man, in which the decidua had so many cells derived from bone marrow primordia. If the sheep's placenta, for example, did not have a contribution from that source, it might not be an appropriate choice for study when the primary object was human. Redman replied that certainly the placenta of the mouse and rat seemed to be different, with cells derived from the bone marrow in the metrial glands. However, to answer the question accurately, one had to have the species-specific markers which so far had not been developed enough to answer the question. He did not think that such markers were available for sheep.

Reference

Ellendorff F, Tyndale-Biscoe CH, Mark R (1988) In: The Endocrine Control of the Fetus (Eds: Künzel W and Jensen A), pp. 193–200. Springer, Berlin.

11

Fetal Amino Acids

I. CETIN, A. M. MARCONI AND G. PARDI

Clinica Ostetrico-Ginecologica, Ospedale San Paolo, Università di Milano, Italy

The supply of amino acids from the umbilical circulation to the growing fetus, and features of both placental and fetal amino acid metabolism, have been studied in animals. Among the various species the sheep has been studied most intensively, principally because it is feasible in this species to catheterize chronically the maternal and fetal circulations. Thus, studies of metabolism and of the transport of amino acids can be carried out under unstressed steady-state conditions. In this species, studies of the uterine and umbilical arterial and venous concentrations of amino acids have demonstrated that there is a large uptake of most neutral and basic amino acids by the pregnant uterus and, similarly, a large uptake of amino acids by the fetus (Lemons et al., 1976; Holzman et al., 1979a). In the normal fetal lamb the uptake of amino acids from the umbilical circulation through the placenta far exceeds the rate of nitrogen accretion, consistent with studies that have shown a fairly high rate of amino acid catabolism and oxidation in the fetus (Battaglia and Meschia, 1986). The rate of fetal nitrogen accretion has also been calculated in a number of different species from measurements of nitrogen concentration in fetuses at different gestational ages (Widdowson et al., 1979; Meier et al., 1981b; Sparks et al., 1985).

Recently, studies of fetal amino acid metabolism have been extended to fetal hepatic metabolism by chronic catheterization of the fetal hepatic vein (Marconi et al., 1989). Using this preparation, umbilical and hepatic arterio-venous concentration differences have been compared. Most amino acids, which enter the umbilical circulation from the placenta, are then taken up by the fetal liver. Glutamate and serine are exceptions in that there is a net hepatic release of these amino acids into the umbilical circulation. Since there is a large fetal hepatic uptake of glutamine and glycine, these observations suggest that glutamate and serine may be synthesized from glutamine and glycine within the fetal liver.

Fetal Autonomy and Adaptation. Edited by G. S. Dawes, A. Zacutti, F. Borruto and A. Zacutti, Jr
© 1990 John Wiley & Sons Ltd

The role of the placenta in metabolizing amino acids, either by catabolism or by transamination and synthesis of some non-essential amino acids, has been suggested by several observations. First is the demonstration that there is a net ammonia production by the placenta, which is delivered into both the uterine and umbilical circulations (Holzman et al., 1977, 1979a, 1979b). Moreover, there is a high activity for the branched-chain amino acid transferase in both human (Jaroszewicz et al., 1971) and sheep (Goodwin et al., 1987) placentas, suggesting a significant metabolism of the branched-chain amino acids to their corresponding alpha-keto acids.

In humans, the concentration of amino acids is higher in fetal than in maternal blood. Such observations are in agreement with a number of studies demonstrating, both in vivo (Page et al., 1957) and in vitro (Enders et al., 1976; Schneider et al., 1979), active transport systems within the placenta. However, the role of the placenta in the metabolism of amino acids and the effect of amino acid metabolism upon amino acid transport has not been studied in man. In human pregnancies, umbilical amino acid concentrations can be studied at the time of delivery, either at caesarean section or at vaginal delivery. More recently, the possibility of sampling fetal blood in vitro from the umbilical vein has made possible the study of fetal amino acid concentrations during intrauterine life at different gestational ages at a time when the fetus is free of the stress of parturition.

Human Studies

At caesarean section, plasma amino acid concentrations are significantly higher in fetal than in maternal blood. Figure 1 presents mean amino acid concentrations in maternal arterial and in umbilical venous plasma of 17 normal pregnancies between 37 and 40 weeks of gestational age. For most amino acids a significant relationship is found between maternal arterial and umbilical venous values.

Many investigators have studied the veno-arterial concentration differences of umbilical amino acids in human fetuses at the time of elective caesarean section (Prenton and Young, 1969; Velazquez et al., 1976; Hayashi et al., 1978; Pohlandt, 1978; Cetin et al., 1988). Figure 2 presents the mean umbilical veno-arterial amino acid concentration differences in 17 normal (AGA) fetuses between 37 and 40 weeks of gestational age. The samples were obtained at the time of elective caesarean section. In normal fetuses, significant umbilical veno-arterial differences are found for most essential amino acids, and there is a significant umbilical veno-arterial difference for total alpha-amino nitrogen (4.16 ± 1.04 mg/l; $p < 0.001$). An estimate of the umbilical uptake of nitrogen by the human fetus can be obtained as follows. The quantification of human umbilical blood flow has been attempted using Doppler ultrasound techniques by analysis of velocity waveforms (Griffin et al., 1983). If we assume an umbilical

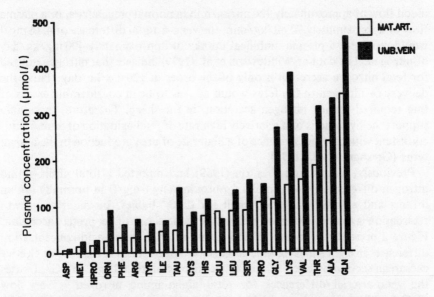

FIGURE 1   Mean plasma amino acid concentrations in the maternal radial artery and in the umbilical vein of normal fetuses between 37 and 40 weeks of gestational age at caesarean section

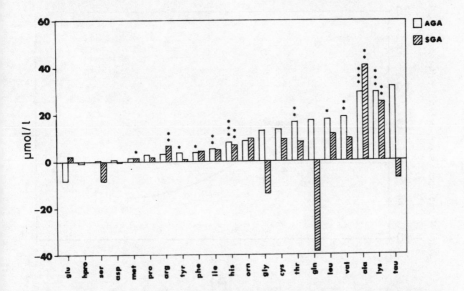

FIGURE 2   Mean umbilical veno-arterial plasma amino acid concentration differences in AGA and SGA fetuses between 37 and 40 weeks of gestational age at caesarean section. Significance of the difference from zero is reported: $* = p < 0.05$; $** = p < 0.01$; $*** = p < 0.001$. From Cetin et al., 1988. Reproduced by permission of C. V. Mosby Co.

blood flow of approximately 120 ml/kg/min in normal pregnancies, or a plasma flow of approximately 70 ml/kg/min, the veno-arterial difference of 4.16 mg/l would represent a plasma umbilical uptake of approximately 400 mg/kg/day of nitrogen. The data of Widdowson et al. (1979) indicate that nitrogen utilized for fetal nitrogen accretion is only of the order of 120 mg/kg/day. Thus, the delivery of nitrogen to the fetus would appear to be in considerable excess of that required for net nitrogen accretion, in the sheep. Therefore, these data support the hypothesis of a relatively high rate of fetal oxidation of amino acids consistent with previous evidence of a high rate of urea production in the human fetus (Gresham et al., 1971).

Previously, Young and Prenton (1969) had reported a total alpha-amino nitrogen difference of 434 μmol/l (approximately 6 mg/l) in normally grown infants and a lower value in 'small for dates' babies. Intrauterine growth retardation is a condition associated with a reduced rate of net protein accretion. Figure 2 presents the mean umbilical veno-arterial amino acid concentration differences in eight small for gestational age (SGA) fetuses at the time of elective caesarean section between 37 and 40 weeks of gestational age. In SGA fetuses the veno-arterial differences for total alpha-amino nitrogen is very low (0.43 ± 2.07 mg/l), and not significantly different from zero. Only methionine,

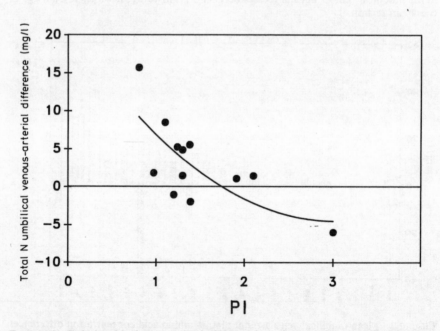

FIGURE 3 Relationship between total alpha-amino nitrogen (N), umbilical venous-arterial difference and pulsatility index (PI) in SGA fetuses between 27 and 40 weeks of gestational age at caesarean section

lysine, histidine, arginine and alanine had significant umbilical veno-arterial concentration differences in these fetuses. Doppler studies of umbilical blood flow velocity waveforms suggest a significant reduction in umbilical blood flow in growth-retarded fetuses (Griffin et al., 1983), which would further reduce the calculated umbilical uptake of amino acids. Thus, it would seem that IUGR pregnancies are associated with a significant reduction in fetal amino acid uptake. Moreover, this finding seems to be correlated with the degree of blood flow impairment. In cases of intrauterine growth retardation the pulsatility index (PI) of the umbilical artery is measured by Doppler examination of flow velocity waveforms. The PI is calculated according to the simplified Gosling formula (Gosling and King, 1974) and reflects changes in pulsatility and peripheral vascular resistance. Figure 3 presents the relationship between the PI and the umbilical veno-arterial difference for total alpha-amino nitrogen in 12 SGA fetuses at elective caesarean section. The lowest umbilical veno-arterial differences were associated with the highest PI, i.e. with the highest blood flow resistances.

Human Studies During Pregnancy

Now that techniques have become available for sampling fetal blood in utero it is possible to study fetal substrate concentrations in a relatively unstressed condition unaffected by parturition and at different gestational ages.

Percutaneous umbilical blood sampling was originally introduced as a technique for sampling fetal blood during the second trimester for prenatal diagnosis (Daffos et al., 1985). In most cases the fetuses are not affected by the disease under study and they can be considered normal. Umbilical venous amino acid concentrations have been measured in normal fetuses during the second trimester by many authors (McIntosh et al., 1984; Kamoun et al., 1985; Soltesz et al., 1985; Cetin et al., 1990). Table 1a presents plasma amino acid concentrations in the umbilical vein of 11 normal fetuses sampled by cordocentesis between 18 and 25 weeks of gestational age. These values are compared to values obtained in 14 normal fetuses sampled at caesarean section between 37 and 40 weeks of gestational age (all values are means ± SE).

The concentrations of most amino acids did not change significantly between the second and third trimester. Significantly lower concentrations were found in the third trimester for methionine, phenylalanine, and tyrosine, while histidine and glycine were significantly higher compared to second trimester fetuses. However, there were no significant changes in total mM concentrations; in the second trimester total mM concentrations are 2.97 ± 0.10 (SE) mM in the third trimester 3.13 ± 0.05 mM.

Maternal 'arterialized' plasma can also be obtained at the time of cordocentesis: maternal total mM concentrations are 1.81 ± 0.05 mM in the

TABLE 1a Umbilical venous amino acid concentrations (μmol/l, $\pm$ SE) in AGA fetuses

	Second trimester	Third trimester	p
Essential			
Val	277.4 ± 14.6	251.1 ± 8.8	NS
Leu	118.0 ± 5.9	133.6 ± 6.1	NS
Ile	67.7 ± 2.9	67.6 ± 3.7	NS
Thr	275.7 ± 22.7	315.8 ± 17.6	NS
Phe	70.3 ± 2.2	60.7 ± 1.8	*
Met	30.3 ± 0.9	24.3 ± 1.1	**
Lys	382.7 ± 25.9	373.6 ± 10.8	NS
His	92.8 ± 8.6	109.6 ± 3.5	*
Arg	73.0 ± 7.2	71.7 ± 7.4	NS
Non-essential			
Gln	448.6 ± 22.3	455.4 ± 20.3	NS
Ala	307.6 ± 11.1	323.9 ± 14.8	NS
Gly	155.0 ± 5.2	257.8 ± 15.6	***
Ser	148.9 ± 6.9	151.8 ± 14.0	NS
Tyr	79.1 ± 4.9	58.9 ± 2.2	***
Orn	98.5 ± 6.5	87.6 ± 7.8	NS
Tau	116.0 ± 6.0	144.0 ± 20.5	NS
Asp	7.1 ± 1.1	10.7 ± 1.4	NS
Glu	46.4 ± 10.5	68.7 ± 13.1	NS
Pro	166.7 ± 16.2	144.1 ± 5.0	NS
H-Pro	36.9 ± 4.2	28.1 ± 0.5	NS

*$p < 0.05$.
**$p < 0.01$.
***$p < 0.001$.

third trimester. Therefore, fetal/maternal molar concentration ratios (F/M ratios) were also not significantly different: 1.66 ± 0.04 in the second trimester and 1.66 ± 0.04 in the third trimester.

Cordocentesis is also used during the third trimester in many centres for the biochemical evaluation of SGA fetuses (Pardi et al., 1987). Since most amino acid concentrations do not change significantly in normal fetuses between the second and the third trimester, SGA fetuses can be compared to AGA fetuses of both trimesters (Cetin et al., 1988).

Table 1b also reports umbilical venous amino acid concentrations from 12 SGA fetuses sampled by cordocentesis between 27 and 39 weeks of gestational age. In SGA fetuses, there is a significant reduction in total alpha-amino nitrogen: 54.0 ± 1.6 mg/l in SGA compared to 63.9 ± 1.1 mg/l in AGA fetuses at term ($p < 0.001$), and to 60.1 ± 2.5 mg/l in AGA fetuses of the second trimester ($p < 0.05$). The three branched-chain amino acids (BCAA), valine, leucine, and isoleucine, are mainly responsible for this reduction. In Figure 4, the sum of the BCAA in the umbilical vein is presented as a function of maternal values.

TABLE 1b Umbilical venous amino acid concentrations (μmol/l, $\pm$ SE) in SGA fetuses

	SGA infants	SGA versus second trimester AGA p	SGA versus third trimester AGA p
Essential			
Val	202.17 $\pm$ 9.16	***	**
Leu	91.83 $\pm$ 5.96	**	***
Ile	51.83 $\pm$ 2.65	**	**
Thr	281.92 $\pm$ 17.71	NS	NS
Phe	65.75 $\pm$ 3.91	NS	NS
Met	21.83 $\pm$ 1.73	***	NS
Lys	310.17 $\pm$ 24.90	*	*
His	93.75 $\pm$ 3.83	NS	*
Arg	61.75 $\pm$ 4.21	NS	NS
Non-essential			
Gln	426.58 $\pm$ 26.25	NS	NS
Ala	290.64 $\pm$ 14.27	NS	NS
Gly	186.42 $\pm$ 8.15	NS	***
Ser	125.17 $\pm$ 5.64	**	**
Tyr	54.83 $\pm$ 4.68	***	NS
Orn	79.75 $\pm$ 5.56	NS	NS
Tau	78.25 $\pm$ 8.60	NS	**
Asp	7.11 $\pm$ 1.82	NS	NS
Glu	52.83 $\pm$ 8.49	NS	NS
Pro	141.08 $\pm$ 5.06	NS	NS
H-Pro	29.67 $\pm$ 9.95	NS	NS

*$p < 0.05$.
**$p < 0.01$.
***$p < 0.001$.

In normal fetuses of the second and third trimester there is a significant correlation between maternal and fetal concentrations, whereas the slope is essentially zero for SGA fetuses, and there is a significant difference both in elevation and in slope from AGA fetuses of both trimesters. At any given maternal concentration, the umbilical venous concentration is lower in SGA fetuses.

The BCAA share a common 'L' transport system in the human placenta (Enders et al., 1976). The differences in umbilical venous concentrations could imply a reduction in the placental transfer of these amino acids. This observation is consistent with a recent study in vitro where the placental uptake of methylamino-isobutyric acid (MeABA) was significantly reduced in SGA compared to AGA pregnancies (Dicke and Henderson, 1988).

Since maternal amino acid concentrations are not different in SGA compared to normal pregnancies, the F/M ratio is significantly reduced in SGA

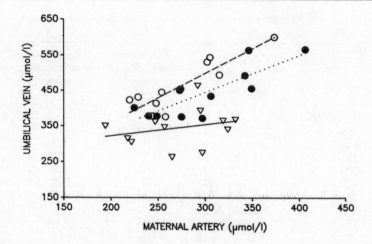

FIGURE 4   Relationship of the sum of the branched-chain amino acids (BCAA) in umbilical venous plasma to maternal arterial values in AGA fetuses of the third trimester (●), of the second trimester (○), and in SGA fetuses (▽). For third trimester AGA: umbilical venous concentration = 126.4 ± 1.1 (maternal arterial concentration); $p < 0.001$, $r = 0.82$. For second trimester AGA: umbilical venous concentration = 77.1 ± 1.4 (maternal arterial concentration); $p < 0.001$; $r = 0.88$. For SGA fetuses the slope is essentially equal to zero. From Cetin et al., 1988; reproduced with permission

pregnancies for most essential amino acids. The F/M total molar concentration ratio for essential alpha-amino nitrogen is 1.43 ± 0.08 in SGA compared to 1.93 ± 0.06 ($p < 0.001$) in AGA of the second trimester and 1.91 ± 0.07 ($p < 0.001$) in AGA of the third trimester.

It is tempting to conclude that the differences found in SGA fetuses are due to altered placental transfer, whether as a reflection of reduced uterine blood flow or from a difference in placental permeability. However, amino acid metabolism may also be altered in these fetuses.

Future Perspectives

There are some questions that still need to be addressed in order to understand fetal amino acid metabolism better.

How are Amino Acids Utilized Within the Fetus?

The first question is related to the fetal and placental utilization of amino acids. The finding that alpha-amino nitrogen is taken up from the umbilical circulation in amounts that exceed the needs for protein accretion suggests that amino acids are utilized during fetal life for other purposes besides protein synthesis. This hypothesis is also supported by the observation of a high rate of urea production by the fetus both in sheep (Gresham et al., 1972) and in human (Gresham et al., 1971) pregnancies. The fetal utilization and oxidation rate of individual amino acids can be estimated directly with the use of tracer methodologies. These studies have been performed in chronically catheterized fetal lambs (Meier et al., 1981a; van Veen et al., 1987). They suggest that the placenta significantly utilizes both leucine and lysine. Moreover, a significant fraction of both lysine and leucine is used within the fetus for oxidative purposes. These points need further demonstration in human pregnancies.

Do the Utilization and Oxidation Rates of Amino Acids Change Under Different Metabolic Conditions?

Another important feature of fetal amino acid metabolism is the question of whether the relative proportions of amino acids utilized for protein synthesis and oxidation by the fetus could change under different metabolic conditions. This point has been addressed in the fetal lamb during maternal fasting. After five days of maternal fasting, glucose umbilical uptake falls to 50% of normal values (Hay et al., 1984), but the total fetal oxygen consumption does not change significantly. In this state of fetal hyperinsulinism, fetal amino acid uptake does not change (Lemons and Schreiner, 1983, 1984), but the rate of urea production increases significantly (Lemons and Schreiner, 1983), suggesting an increase in the utilization of amino acids for oxidation. Leucine tracer studies have shown that although the utilization rate of this amino acid does not change significantly, the fraction of leucine oxidized within the fetus increases significantly during maternal fasting (van Veen et al., 1987). Therefore, there appears to be a redistribution in the relative utilization of leucine for protein synthesis and for oxidation during maternal fasting. In the human fetus under conditions of maternal denutrition or in intrauterine growth retardation, fetal amino acid metabolism might change as well.

How are Amino Acids Transferred and Utilized in Growth-Retarded Fetuses?

In SGA fetuses, the rate of growth is reduced in comparison to normal fetuses. In these fetuses there is a reduction in the delivery of alpha-amino nitrogen through the umbilical circulation. However, in the most severe cases, there is also the possibility that amino acids are no longer used for protein synthesis, but mainly for oxidative purposes.

Therefore, there are two major questions to be answered in SGA fetuses:

1. Is there an alteration in placental transfer for the essential amino acids and in particular for the BCAA?
2. Is the growth-retarded fetus not only not growing but also in a state of net protein catabolism?

The possible role of both pathogenetic mechanisms in fetal growth retardation could be studied with stable isotope methodologies in human pregnancies. Stable isotopes have been used in human pregnancies mainly for the study of maternal glucose metabolism. Amino acids labelled with ^{13}C can be infused in the mother prior to fetal sampling by cordocentesis. The quantity of the tracer that is transferred from the mother to the fetus is an indicator of the placental transfer. Moreover, the dilution of the enrichment of ^{13}C for the amino acid under study in the fetal compartment is an indicator of the relative proportion of fetal catabolism.

Future Treatment

Nutritional supplementation via amniotic injections has been tried in human pregnancies (Heller, 1974; Renaud et al., 1974; Saling et al., 1974; Massobrio et al., 1975). However, the concentration of injected amino acids decreases very rapidly in amniotic fluid. Estimates of portal uptake of nutrients in the fetal lamb show a net consumption of nutrients by the gastrointestinal tract rather than a net absorption (Charlton et al., 1979). Therefore, intra-amniotic injections do not represent a normal route of fetal nutrition.

Nutritional supplementation via intravascular administration of nutrients has been attempted in fetal lambs (Charlton and Johengen, 1987). In a group of experimentally induced growth-retarded fetal lambs, supplemented fetuses appeared to grow at a much higher rate than non-supplemented fetuses. The supplemented fetuses also presented a very big placenta when compared to normal controls.

However, in normal fetuses, not enough knowledge is available on the relative quantities of nutrients needed by the growing fetus. In a state of hypoxia, these nutrients could even prove toxic for brain development. More studies, both in animals and in humans, are needed in order to clarify fetal amino acid requirements for the treatment in future, by nutritional supplementation, of growth-retarded fetuses.

References

Battaglia FC and Meschia G (1986) Fetal and placental metabolism. Part II. Amino acids and lipids. In: An Introduction to Fetal Physiology (Eds: Battaglia FC and Meschia G), pp 100–135. Academic Press: Orlando, Florida.

Cetin I, Marconi AM, Bozzetti P, Sereni LP, Corbetta C, Pardi G, Battaglia FC (1988) Umbilical amino acid concentrations in appropriate and small for gestation age infants: a biochemical difference present in utero. Am J Obstet Gynecol 158: 120–126.

Cetin I, Corbetta C, Sereni LP, Marconi AM, Bozzetti P, Pardi G, Battaglia FC (1990) Umbilical amino acid concentrations in normal and growth retarded fetuses sampled in utero by cordocentesis. Am J Obstet Gynecol 162: 253–261.

Charlton VE and Johengen M (1987) Fetal intravenous nutritional supplementation ameliorates the development of embolization-induced growth retardation in sheep. Pediatr Res 22: 55–61.

Charlton VE, Reis BL, Lofgren DJ (1979) Consumption of carbohydrates, amino acids and oxygen across the intestinal circulation in the fetal sheep. J Dev Physiol 1: 329.

Daffos F, Capella-Pavlovsky M, Forestier F (1985) Fetal blood sampling during pregnancy with use of a needle guided by ultrasound: a study of 606 consecutive cases. Am J Obstet Gynecol 153: 655–660.

Dicke JM and Henderson GI (1988) Placental amino acid uptake in normal and complicated pregnancies. Am J Med Sci 295: 223–227.

Enders RH, Judd RM, Donohue TM, Smith CH (1976) Placental amino acid uptake. III. Transport systems for neutral amino acids. Am J Physiol 230: 706–710.

Goodwin GW, Gibboney W, Paxton R, Harris RA, Lemons JA (1987) Activities of branched-chain aminotransferase and branched-chain 2-oxo acid dehydrogenase complex in tissues of maternal and fetal sheep. Biochem J 242: 305–308.

Gosling RG and King DH (1974) Continuous wave ultrasound as an alternative and complement to x-rays in vascular examinations. In: Cardiovascular Applications of Ultrasound (Ed: Reneman RS), pp. 266–282. North Holland Publishing Company, Amsterdam.

Gresham EL, Simons PS, Battaglia FC (1971) Maternal-fetal urea concentration difference in man: metabolic significance. J Pediatrics 79: 809–811.

Gresham EL, James EJ, Raye JR, Battaglia FC, Makowski EL, Meschia G (1972) Production and excretion of urea by the fetal lamb. Pediatrics 50: 372–379.

Griffin D, Cohen-Ovebeek T, Campbell S (1983) Fetal and utero-placental blood flow. Clinics in Obstet & Gynecol 10: 565–602.

Hay WW Jr, Sparks JW, Wilkening RB, Battaglia FC, Meschia G (1984) Fetal glucose uptake and utilization as functions of maternal glucose concentration. Am J Physiol 246: E237–E242.

Hayashi S, Sanada K, Sagawa N, Yamada N, Kido K (1978) Umbilical vein-artery differences of plasma amino acids in the last trimester of human pregnancy. Biol Neonate 34: 11–18.

Heller L (1974) Intrauterine amino acid feeding of the fetus. In: Parenteral Nutrition in Infancy and Childhood (Eds: Bode H and Warshaw J), p. 206. Plenum Press, New York.

Holzman IR, Lemons JA, Meschia G, Battaglia FC (1977) Ammonia production by the pregnant uterus. Proc Soc Exp Biol & Med 156: 27–30.

Holzman IR, Lemons JA, Meschia G, Battaglia FC (1979a) Uterine uptake of amino acids and glutamine-glutamate balance across the placenta of the pregnant ewe. J Dev Physiol 1: 137–149.

Holzman IR, Philipps AF, Battaglia FC (1979b) Glucose metabolism and ammonia production by the human placenta in vitro. Pediatric Res 13: 117–120.

Jaroszewicz L, Jozwik M, Jaroszewicz K (1971) The activity of aminotransferases in human placenta in early pregnancy. Biochem Med 5: 436–439.

Kamoun P, Droin V, Forestier F, Daffos F (1985) Free amino acids in human fetal plasma. Clin Chim Acta 150: 227–230.

Lemons JA and Schreiner RL (1983) Amino acid metabolism in the ovine fetus. Am J Physiol 244: E459–E466.

Lemons JA and Schreiner RL (1984) Metabolic balance of the ovine fetus during the fed and fasted states. Annals of Nutrition and Metabolism 28: 268–280.

Lemons JA, Adcock EW III, Jones MD Jr, Naughton MA, Meschia G, Battaglia FC (1976) Umbilical uptake of amino acids in the unstressed fetal lamb. J Clin Invest 58: 1428–1434.

Marconi AM, Battaglia FC, Meschia G, Sparks JW (1989) A comparison of amino acid arteriovenous differences across the placenta and liver in the fetal lamb. Am J Physiol 257: E909–915.

Massobrio M, Margaria E, Campogravide M et al. (1975) Treatment of severe feto-placental insufficiency by means of intraamniotic injection of amino acids. In: Therapy of Feto-Placental Insufficiency (Ed: Salvadori B), p. 296. Springer-Verlag, Berlin.

McIntosh N, Rodeck CH, Heath R (1984) Plasma amino acids of the mid-trimester human fetus. Biol Neonate 45: 218–224.

Meier PR, Peterson RB, Bonds DR, Meschia G, Battaglia FC (1981a) Rates of protein synthesis and turnover in fetal life. Am J Physiol 240: E320–E324.

Meier PR, Teng C, Battaglia FC, Meschia G (1981b) The rate of amino acid nitrogen and total nitrogen accumulation in the fetal lamb. Proc Soc Exp Biol & Med 167: 463–468.

Page EW, Glendening MB, Margolis A, Harper HA (1957) Transfer of D- and L-histidine across the human placenta. Am J Obstet Gynecol 73: 589–594.

Pardi G, Buscaglia M, Ferrazzi E, Bozzetti P, Marconi AM, Cetin I, Battaglia FC, Makowski EL (1987) Cord sampling for the evaluation of oxygenation and acid-base balance in growth-retarded human fetuses. Am J Obstet Gynecol 157: 1221–1228.

Pohlandt F (1978) Plasma amino acid concentrations in umbilical cord vein and artery of newborn infants after elective caesarean section or spontaneous delivery. J Pediatr 92: 617–623.

Prenton MA and Young M (1969) Umbilical vein-artery and uterine arterio-venous plasma amino acids differences. J Obstet Gynaecol Br Commonw 76: 404–411.

Renaud R, Kirschtetter L, Koehl C et al. (1974) Amino acid intraamniotic injection. In: Recent Progress in Obstetrics and Gynecology. Proceedings of the Seventh World Congress of Obstetrics and Gynecology (Eds: Persianinov L, Chervakova T, Presl J), p. 234. Excerpta Medica, Prague.

Saling E, Dudenhausen J, Kynast G (1974) Basic investigations about compensatory nutrition of the malnourished fetus. In: Recent Progress in Obstetrics and Gynecology. Proceedings of the Seventh World Congress in Obstetrics and Gynecology (Eds: Persianinov L, Chervakova T, Presl J), p. 227. Excerpta Medica, Prague.

Schneider H, Mohlen KH, Challier JC, Dancis J (1979) Transfer of glutamic acid across the human placenta perfused in vitro. Br J Obstet Gynecol 86: 229–306.

Soltesz G, Harris D, MacKenzie IZ, Aynsley-Green A (1985) The metabolic and endocrine milieu of the human fetus and mother at 19–21 weeks of gestation. I. Plasma amino acid concentrations. Pediatr Res 19: 92–93.

Sparks JW, Girard JR, Callikan S, Battaglia FC (1985) Growth of the fetal guinea pig: physical and chemical characteristics. Am J Physiol 248: E132–E139.

van Veen LCP, Teng C, Hay WW Jr, Meschia S, Battaglia FC (1987) Leucine disposal and oxidation rates in the fetal lamb. Metabolism 36: 48–53.

Velazquez A, Rosado A, Bernal A, Noriega L, Arevalo N (1976) Amino acid pools in the feto-maternal system. Biol Neonate 29: 28–40.

Widdowson EM, Southgate DAT, Hey EN (1979) Body composition of the fetus and infant. In: Nutrition and Metabolism of the Fetus and Infant (Ed: Visser HKA). Fifth Nutricia Symposium, pp. 169–177. Martinus Nijhoff, The Hague.

Young M and Prenton MA (1969) Maternal and fetal plasma amino acid concentrations during gestation and in retarded fetal growth. J Obstet Gynaecol Br Commonw 76: 333–344.

Discussion

Patrick was intrigued to learn that in man, as in sheep, the placenta can, so to say, catabolize the fetus. Cetin explained that this had happened only in three of her 11 cases, sectioned electively at 37–40 weeks gestation and with severe growth retardation (all below the 2nd centile) and with a poor prognosis. She had no further information from ultrasound studies on these fetuses. More data were required on their behaviour, and also on better indices of protein catabolism, such as might be obtained by measurement of 3-methyl histidine, hydroxyproline and urea.

Thornburg wondered whether there had been a change in the numbers of receptors for or binding of amino acids. Cetin replied that Dicke and Henderson (1988) had studied leucine and methylaminoisobutyric acid (MeAIB) transport in the placenta in vitro. In this study, placental uptake of MeAIB by vesicles isolated from the villous membrane of the syncytiotrophoblast was found to be significantly reduced in pregnancies complicated by intrauterine growth retardation when compared to normal pregnancies. Glycine was of special interest because, though the smallest amino acid with MW = 75, it does not 'pass through' the placenta in animal studies (unpublished data). There was as yet no evidence on receptor numbers.

Simpson pointed out that low-density lipoprotein, a major source of cholesterol for the formation of placental progesterone, must be a potential source of amino acids in the placenta, and hence could dilute the isotope which Cetin had infused. Cetin agreed that this was possible. However, she found it extraordinary that, when labelled serine was infused into the fetal lamb, glycine also was enriched (unpublished data). It was astonishing that 90% of fetal glycine was derived from serine, presumably in the placenta or fetal liver, releasing a carbon atom as methylenetetrahydrofolate. The 1-carbon atom derived from serine and carried by tetrahydrofolate can be transferred to various acceptor molecules and can be used for incorporation into DNA. The placenta certainly metabolized proteins rapidly, since Battaglia had shown a large increase in placental amino acids with elapse of time between the death of a sheep and placental extraction (personal communication).

Amino Acid Transport and Umbilical Blood Flow

Hanson enquired whether the transport of amino acids was related to umbilical flow; if indeed the pulsatility index (PI) could be regarded as a reliable measure of flow. Cetin replied that the PI was related to the umbilical nitrogen arteriovenous (A-V) difference but not to the concentration of amino acids in the umbilical vein. The change in A-V difference was due to a *rise* in arterial concentration. She said that the fetuses with the highest PI did not appear to have the least transport across the placenta, as judged by umbilical venous concentrations.

Dawes wondered whether the growth-retarded fetus had been using amino acids as an energy source, as well as having the placenta steal amino acids. Did this mean that such fetuses lost protein from the liver, or the brain? Pardi did not know. He pointed out that the oxygen content and glucose concentration in the umbilical vein was normal. In Robinson's experiments in growth-retarded sheep the flow of O_2 and glucose to the fetus was still appropriate to fetal weight even when they were losing amino acids. If a particular marker for amino acid availability was required he would advise measuring the concentration of the branched-chain amino acids. Simpson added that the insulin/glucocorticoid ratio might be considered as a marker of net protein metabolism.

Markers of Fetal Deterioration

Dawes reverted to the need for measures of fetal health in clinical practice. If the placenta steals amino acids from the grossly growth-retarded fetus, is the clinical principle of keeping that fetus in utero if possible at 28 weeks, well-founded? In that case oxygen enrichment of the maternal inspired air might be pointless? Do such infants really do well postnatally? Redman replied that there were rare cases in which abdominal girth declined in utero, in fetuses which already had other signs of distress. This was an example of extreme terminal decompensation. It was highly desirable to obtain exact measurements of the time course of this process; perhaps it would be possible using the fetal lamb. Cetin agreed that it was very difficult to study the natural history of fetal deterioration in man, since the amino acid V-A difference was not available before delivery. Pardi spoke of the hazard of cordocentesis in such infants, with the occasional appearance of bradycardia after taking an umbilical arterial blood sample in utero. He did not regard it as safe to take an arterial sample; it was less risky to take a venous sample when cordocentesis was necessary. Sampling both vessels at the same time to measure the V-A amino acid gradient in utero would be dangerous.

Reference

Dicke JM and Henderson GI (1988) Am J Med Sci 295: 223–227.

12

Development of the Fetal Neuroendocrine Brain for Adaptation

F. ELLENDORFF, R. GROSSMANN, N. MILEWSKI,
M. KLEMPT AND E. MA

Institut für Kleintierzucht, Celle, Bundesforschungsanstalt für Landwirtschaft (FAL),
3100 Celle, West Germany

Amongst the homeostatic mechanisms essential to prenatal and postnatal survival are those of fluid and electrolyte balance, such as the hypothalamo-neurohypophyseal system and the hypothalamo-pituitary-adrenal system. Extensive research has yielded considerable information on the prenatal control of both systems, yet major gaps persist. For example, the initiation of system control and the step-by-step ontogeny of differentiation and maturation is far from being elucidated. It is of paramount importance to comprehend the onset of expression of peptide genes within endocrine active neurones and other cells. It is equally important to know how gene expression relates to function, and eventually to the maintenance of homeostasis and the ability to adapt to changing environmental conditions. Finally, common principles that are recognised across the diversity of species, or in species with specific genetic traits, may help to apply knowledge not only to particular species but to the human as well.

The following contribution consists of a comparative approach to the hypothalamo-neurohypophyseal system, in particular to the onset and further ontogeny of arginine vasotocin and lysine vasopressin in the chick embryo and pig fetus, respectively (see also: Ellendorff and Grossman, 1988; Ellendorff et al., 1990; Milewski et al., 1989; Sander-Richter et al., 1987; Grossman and Ellendorff, 1986a, 1986b; Weindl et al;. 1984). In addition, the paper will deal with some preliminary findings related to prenatal POMC-gene expression in the pig fetal pituitary and brain. POMC (pro-opiomelanocortin) is the

Fetal Autonomy and Adaptation. Edited by G. S. Dawes, A. Zacutti, F. Borruto and A. Zacutti, Jr
©1990 John Wiley & Sons Ltd

precursor molecule of ACTH and endogenous opioids that are part of homeostatic and adaptive mechanisms.

The Hypothalamo-Neurohypophyseal System
in the Chick Embryo (21 days of incubation)

The hypothalamo-neurohypophyseal system appears at about day 2 (40–45 h) of incubation, when the formation of the posterior pituitary becomes visible (Freeman and Vince, 1974). The central nervous system is then in the course of neural tube closure and hindbrain differentiation. For comparison, on embyronal day 4 the first active movements of the head and the cochlear nucleus are seen. But there is still no mRNA expression for AVT/MT (arginine vasotocin/mesotocin) anywhere in the neural tissue (Milewski et al., 1989). On day 6 of incubation, when the retinal nerves have just reached the optic tract and the eyelids are about to move, the first AVT/MT mRNA signal originates in the PVN (paraventricular nucleus). A 39-mer oligonucleotide, complementary to the base sequence of AVT, was used. The homology was about 80–90%, indicating that AVT is not fully distinguishale from MT. At day 6 the signal is still weak and diffuse, with silver granules covering only a few cells. Indeed only dark-field microscopy provided convincing evidence of signal intensity above background. No signal was detectable in the supraoptic nucleus (SON) or in other brain structures. Six days later, on day 12, the size of the brain is near doubled. The signal in the PVN has spread out, and the SON displays hydridizing activity. Around the same time (day 11–14) the appearance of neurosecretory material has been described with more conventional techniques (Bock et al., 1968; Lawzewitsch, 1969). Two days later (embryonal day 14), the system has grown more complex; positive signals spread in large patterns over the hypothalamus. This process appears to reach a plateau by day 16, since it is hardly distinguishable from that on day 18. In fact, comparison with immunohistochemical patterns of distribution within the HNS (hypothalamo-neurophyseal system) in the adult (Viglietti-Panzica and Contenti, 1983) shows little difference to the embryo at day 18. Using in situ hybridization, two apparently different cell types appeared on day 18, one that expressed the AVT/MT signal weakly, the other strongly. Both cell types are only located periventricularly.

Although these findings, and those of others (Mosier, 1955; Blähser and Heinrichs, 1982; Tennyson et al., 1986), point to the early presence of AVT/MT activities, the regulation of the onset of AVT/MT biosynthesis is uncertain.

Another area that remains poorly investigated is the functional implication of the presence of neurosecretory material. For example, the first time at which the pituitary of the chick embryo contains vasopressin (antidiuretic) activity is day 9 of embryonal development (Wingstrand, 1954). When AVT was given on day 12 kidney water reabsorption was altered (Murphy et al., 1981).

Plasma AVT levels appear to exceed baseline around day 16 (Klempt et al., 1989), but only from day 18 has the embryo's response to hyperosmotic stimulation been tested. There is a large gap from the time when the first urine secretion from the mesonephros is reported (day 4 or 5 of embryonal development; Gruenwald, 1952) or from the time when the secretory tubules of the metanephros and glomeruli are present structurally and functionally around day 11 (Romanoff, 1967).

Finally, an important indication of the maturation and functional integrity of the hypothalamo-neurohypophyseal system would be derived from analysis of action potential traffic along axons that originate in the magnocellular system and terminate in the posterior pituitary. This is most likely the pathway taken by the neurosecretory products from magnocellular neurones to the posterior pituitary. In recent years (Grossmann and Ellendorff, 1986a, 1986b) it has become evident that, during late embryonal development (day 17 to hatching on day 21), obvious progressive changes occur. The number of spontaneously active neurones increases, the action potential width diminishes, and the conduction velocity increases simultaneously. All this indicates that even in the later stages of prenatal development the HNS has not reached maturity. We need to link neural activity to changes in plasma osmolality. Further, it will be necessary to relate maturation of the HNS-AVT system to the control of functions such as water balance, cardiovascular functions, behaviour, adrenal activity, or neuromodulatory processes.

The Pig Fetus (114 days of gestation)

The other species to be discussed is the pig. Here knowledge of the prenatal development of the HNS is even less than in the chick. All we know is the time of onset of gene expression for lysine vasopressin (LVP mRNA; Milewski, 1989) and of immunohistochemical evidence for the LVP-carrier molecule (Stimmer et al., 1988). There is a considerable difference between the two; while part of the carrier molecule is immunohistochemically detectable by day 25 of fetal development, gene expression for LVP only appears on day 40.

There is no explanation for this discrepancy. It may be due to technical limitations, but it may also have other unknown biological reasons. Unlike the chick embryo, in which the first mRNA signal for neurohypophyseal hormones appears in the PVN, the SON is the site of LVP mRNA origin in the pig. Oxytocin mRNA appears 1–2 days later, again in the SON. Both peptide signals are present in the paraventricular nucleus of the pig fetus on day 44. Thus by little more than 1/3 of pregnancy (duration 114 days) LVP is expressed in both major neurosecretory structures of the hypothalamus.

These findings do not yield evidence for a role of LVP in the control of water balance or other LVP-related homeostatic phenomena. In the pig this has only been studied in the later stages of development, relative to the onset of gene expression, probably because there is then easier access to the fetus. Thus, LVP can be detected around day 80 in fetal plasma, but it is present at an earlier age. Already on day 60 the posterior pituitary is loaded with immunoreactive neurophysin. It is also known that LVP, given to the 80-day-old fetus, increases urine osmolality (Stanier, 1972) indicating that kidney function is present at this time and probably that receptors for LVP are active. A dramatic, well-known but unspecific stimulator of AVP release—uterine clamping—enhances LVP discharge on day 90—the earliest time tested (Forsling et al., 1979). A 20% haemorrhagic stimulus (probably less traumatic) clearly elevates plasma LVP from day 109, while at earlier stages, i.e. day 107 or less, the responses are less convincing (MacDonald et al., 1986).

Thus, despite a general paucity of information, we have a few indicators to orientate research in the pig fetus, with a large catalogue of questions to answer. Some need to address the regulation of the onset of gene expression, as in the chick embryo and other species. Others concern the gap between the onset of gene expression and the first time the peptide is sent down the axon into the posterior pituitary and/or into the circulation or released into the environment of the neurosecretory neurone. We know neither its function there nor the controlling mechanisms. Of equal importance are questions as to the functions of VP in prenatal life. Must we limit our thoughts to the classical functions of VP on water reabsorption in the kidney, on the control of the cardiovascular system or on behaviour, or should we consider less conventional tasks such as neurogenic or morphogenic activity in the HNS or elsewhere? These questions have not yet been addressed. Little, if anything, is known of the ontogeny of AVP receptors during prenatal life, of controlling or interfering neurotransmitters (including neuropeptides), which may or may not resemble those in the adult. For example, endogenous opioid peptides participate as regulators of hormone release in the posterior lobe. If this is so in the fetus, then the in situ opiate synthesizing machinery must develop prenatally. In the pig in situ hybridization detects proencephalin-B in the fetal brain from around day 34 (Pittius et al., 1987). Immunoreactive β-endorphin is also present from day 34 onwards.

Recently, in the pig (Ma et al., unpublished observations), we demonstrated POMC (pro-opiomelanocortin) in the pituitary as early as day 30 of fetal life. Since this is the precursor molecule not only for the opiate family but also for ACTH, it may be that ACTH is also present in early fetal life. Thus the HNS and pituitary-adrenal system may participate in early fetal homeostatic and adaptive functions.

There is no doubt that, for all species investigated and in particular for the human, we are still far away from full understanding of prenatal development of homeostatic and adaptive functions and their control.

References

Blähser S and Heinrichs M (1982) Immunoreactive neuropeptide systems in avian embryos (domestic mallard, domestic fowl, Japanese quail). Cell Tiss Res 223: 287–303.

Bock R, Brinkmann H, Maschwort W (1968) Färberische Beobachtungen zur Frage nach dem primären Bildungsort von Neurosekret im supraoptico-hypophysären System. Zeitschr f Zellforschung 87: 543.

Ellendorff F and Grossmann R (1984) Functional ontogeny of neurons in the chick embryo. Res Perinatal Med (II) 2: 13.

Ellendorff F and Grossmann R (1988) Development of neuroendocrine pathways of the hypothalamo-neurohypophysial system (HNS) in the prenatal chick and pig. In: Fetal and Neonatal Development (Ed: Jones CT) Vol 7, S213–219.

Ellendorff F, Grossmann R, Milewski N, Klempt M, Ma E (1990) Development of the Fetal Neuroendocrine Brain (in press).

Forsling ML, Macdonald AA, Ellendorff F (1979) The neurohypophyseal hormones. Anim Reprod Sc 2: 43–56.

Freemann BM and Vince MA (1974) Development of the Avian Embryo. Chapman and Hall, London.

Grossmann R and Ellendorff F (1986a) Functional development of the prenatal brain. I. Recording of extracellular action potentials from the magnocellular system of the 18-day-old chicken embryo. Exp Brain Res 62: 635–641.

Grossmann R and Ellendorff F (1986b) Functional development of the prenatal brain. II. Ontogeny of the hypothalamo-neurophysial axis in the pre- and perinatal chicken brain. Exp Brain Res 62: 642–647.

Gruenwald P (1952) Development of the excretory system. Ann N.Y. Acad Sci 55: 142–146.

Klempt M, Ellendorff F, Grossmann R (1989) Origin of secretory activity of magnocellular hypothalamic neurons in vivo. Acta Endocrinologica (Suppl) 120: 248.

Lawzewitsch von I (1969) Development of the neurosecretory hypothalamic-hypophyseal system of the chick embryo as evidenced in the total preparation. Acta Anat 72: 83–93.

Macdonald AA, Forsling ML, Ellendorff F, Beermann U (1986) Effect of haemorrhage on plasma lysine vasopressin and the cardiovascular responses to vasopressin in the pig fetus. Quart J Exp Physiol 71: 267–275.

Milewski N (1989) Beginn und Entwicklung des Expression von Peptidhormongenen während der Fötalentwicklung im Hypothalamo-neurohypophysären System bei Huhn und Schwein. Dissertation, Universität Göttingen.

Milewski N, Ivell R, Grossmann R, Ellendorff F (1989) Embryonal development of arginine vasotocin/mesotocin gene expression in the chicken brain. J Neuroendocrin 1: 473–483.

Mosier HD (1955) The development of the hypothalamo-neurophyseal secretory system in the chick embryo. Endocrin 57: 661–669.

Murphy MJ, Brown SC, Brown PS (1981) Arginine vasotocin and osmoregulation during embryonic chick development. Amer Zool 21: 913.

Pittius CW, Ellendorff F, Höllt V, Parvizi N (1987) Ontogenetic development of proenkephalin A and proenkephalin B messenger RNA in fetal pigs. Exp Brain Res 69: 208–212.

Romanoff AL (1967) Biochemistry of the Avian Embryo. Wiley, New York.

Sander-Richter H, Schams D, Ellendorff F (1987) Fetal and postnatal oxytocin secretion in the pig before and after a prostaglandin challenge. J Dev Physiol 10: 63.

Stanier MW (1972) Development of intra-renal solute gradients in fetal and post-natal life. Pflügers Arch 336: 263–270.

Stimmer H, Weindl A, Bruhn T, Parvizi N, Ellendorff F (1988) The fetal and neonatal development of the hypothalamo-neurohypophyseal neurosecretory system of the pig brain. In: Fetal and Neonatal Development (Ed: Jones CT), pp. 254–257. Perinatology Press, New York.

Tennyson VM, Nilaver G, Hou-Yu A, Valiquette G, Zimmermann EA (1986) Immunocytochemical study of the development of vasotocin/mesotocin in the hypothalamo-hypophyseal system of the chick embryo. Cell Tiss Res 243: 15–31.

Viglietti-Panzica C and Contenti E (1983) Cytodifferentiation of the paraventricular nucleus in the chick embryo: a golgi and electron-microscopy study. Cell and Tiss Res 229: 281–297.

Weindl A, Bruhn T, Parvizi N (1984) Ontogeny of neurohypophyseal peptide containing neurons in the pig brain. In: Fetal Neuroendocrinology (Eds: Ellendorff F, Gluckman P, Parvizi N), pp. 35–38. Perinatalogy Press, New York.

Wingstrand KG (1954) Neurosecretion and antidiuretic activity in chick embryo with remarks on the subcommissural organ. Arkiv Zool 6: 41–67.

Discussion

In reply to questions, Ellendorff explained that in the pig vasopressin is expressed in the hypothalamus fairly early, i.e. around day 41/42 of fetal life, but functional activity was not detected before 90–95 days. However, activity was not sought earlier than 80 days. Opiate receptors were present much earlier, but evidence of function had not yet been sought before 100 days, when microinjection of β-endorphin inhibited LH secretion.

Dawes referred to the evidence of Anand et al. (1988) which showed that opiate receptors must be present and functional by 28 weeks gestation in man, since fentanyl blocked the rise in plasma catecholamines and corticosteroids, when given to infants undergoing surgery to tie a patent ductus arteriosus (under nitrous oxide and with neuromuscular blockade). There was no earlier evidence.

Ellendorff could not imagine that gene expression could occur without giving rise to function of biological importance. But there was doubt expressed as to whether this was certain. Challis wondered whether gene expression was at once translated into functional peptides. He was, for example, concerned about interpreting slot blots of POMC mRNA in the sheep pituitary, between 100 and 145 days gestation, because of the high background noise and small signal (McMillen et al., 1988).

Dawes wished to know how physiological control was effected before general release of hormones such as catecholamines or ACTH into the circulation. Was there fetal adaptation before, say 90 days gestation? Fetuses were said to survive hypoxia astonishingly well before that. How good was that evidence? and did it depend on cell-to-cell interaction? However, Ellendorff's primary concern was with the control of normal development. He speculated that vasopressin, when it first appeared, might not display its classic physiological functions, but neural pathfinding or differentiation of neural tissue for example. The LH gene is expressed on day 40 in the pig. If the fetus is stimulated with GNRH on day 55–60 there is no response in pituitary LH, in the pig, even though, due to intravenous injection of GnRH it reaches the pituitary. So there is a time gap of 20 days at least.

To a question from Challis as to what turns on gene expression, Ellendorff replied that he did not know. He thought of trying a (classic) osmotic stimulus. Simpson wondered whether an external signal was necessary; perhaps gene expression was simply a consequence of a timed intracellular program, though, he confessed, that only pushed the question further back.

Application to Man

The subsequent discussion showed the difficulty of applying these ideas to human material. Pardi pointed out that normal early human fetal tissue was available from abortions. With ethical approval and good will it could be made available for research purposes. Visser remarked that function, as shown by fetal muscle movements, could be observed from 7 weeks gestation in man.

Ellendorff replied that in the chick embryo staining of brain sections indicated neurosecretory material as early as day 4 of embryonic life, but there was no evidence of AVT/MT mRNA before day 6. In the pig such changes in the posterior pituitary were not visible histologically by day 18, but were present by day 25; however, in situ hybridization does not provide an mRNA signal for vasopressin or oxytocin before day 41/42. It was doubtful whether such differences could be established from human observations. And indeed to Ellendorf the presence of a limb-bud was a relatively late stage of differentiation, whereas to Visser this was early, since movement could not yet be detected. Animal studies were already far ahead in this field.

References

Anand KJS, Sippell WG, Aynsley-Green A (1988) Lancet i: 62–65.
McMillen IC, Mercer JE, Thorburn GD (1988) J Mol Endocrinol 1: 141–145.

13

Perinatal Asphyxic Brain Damage—the Potential for Therapeutic Intervention

C. E. WILLIAMS, P. D. GLUCKMAN, A. J. GUNN,
W. K. TAN AND M. DRAGUNOW
Department of Paediatrics, University of Auckland, Auckland,
New Zealand

While the precise relationships between perinatal asphyxia and subsequent neurological disabilities are uncertain, it is generally accepted that perinatal asphyxia is a major cause of perinatal death, cerebral palsy, and associated cognitive disorders (Mulligan et al., 1980; Hill and Volpe, 1982; Freeman, 1985; Volpe and Hill, 1987; Robertson et al., 1989). Perinatal asphyxial insults may occur either prepartum, intrapartum, or neonatally (Low et al., 1989): however, increasingly it is recognized that asphyxial encephalopathies often result from prenatal insults (Bejar et al., 1988). Despite the successes of modern obstetrical practice with increasing use of physiological fetal monitoring during labour, there is clearly a place for additional therapeutic approaches.

Sufficient progress has been made in understanding the mechanisms underlying hypoxic-ischaemic-induced neuronal death to suggest that therapeutic intervention is conceptually possible at two points. Firstly, for a fetus known to be at high risk, prophylactic agents may increase the resistance of neurones to asphyxia. Secondly, having identified that an asphyxic episode has occurred, intervention may reduce delayed neuronal death and promote recovery of the brain. In this paper we shall review current concepts of neuronal death, the pathogenesis of perinatal hypoxic-ischaemic encephalopathy, and possible strategies for therapeutic intervention. Recent experimental data suggest that reduction of neurological morbidity during the perinatal period may eventually be possible.

Fetal Autonomy and Adaptation. Edited by G. S. Dawes, A. Zacutti, F. Borruto and A. Zacutti, Jr
© 1990 John Wiley & Sons Ltd

Mechanisms of Asphyxia-Induced Neuronal Death

Several interacting processes appear to lead to necrotic cell death during or following an asphyxial insult (Siesjo, 1981; Rothman and Olney, 1987; Choi, 1988). These processes share a final common pathway of loss of plasma membrane integrity, cell lysis and death (Dean, 1987; Van der Vusse et al., 1989). Osmotic forces and swelling are thought to contribute to the loss of membrane integrity (Steenburgen and Jennings, 1984; Rothman and Olney, 1987). Both in vitro and in vivo studies suggest three phases of neuronal death related to an isolated insult. Firstly, during the acute period there may be 'primary' neuronal death; then after relief from the insult there may be a phase of 'reactive' neuronal death; thirdly, 'delayed' neuronal death (Kirino, 1982; Pulsinelli et al., 1982) may occur some hours or days after the insult. Generally, the severity of the insult affects the time course of the cell death: moderate insults trigger delayed death, whereas the more severe insults can lead to primary cell death (Rothman and Olney, 1987).

Primary Neuronal Death

Asphyxia per se leads to energy failure causing depolarization of neurones, and loss of many important energy-dependent homeostatic mechanisms. This loss of ion homeostasis leads to osmotic influxes of water with increases in intracellular volume that can lead to lysis and cell death (Rothman and Olney, 1987). During an insult extracellular potassium and the excitotoxic amino acids glutamate and aspartate accumulate (Benveniste et al., 1984) both because of failure of re-uptake and also increased release. These favour further depolarization of adjacent neurones, apparent as spreading depolarization.

In lower concentrations the excitatory amino acids have different effects. Acting through postsynaptic NMDA receptors and the associated calcium conductance channels, excitotoxic activity leads to an influx of calcium into neurones. With further calcium entry through voltage dependent channels and failure of the energy-dependent processes of Ca^{2+} sequestration and removal by the Na^+ Ca^{2+} pump, calcium accumulates intracellularly (Uematsu et al., 1988) and activates calcium-dependent processes leading to further injury.

Reactive Cell Death

During re-oxygenation following an insult several poorly defined events may occur. Hypoxanthine, a degradation product of ATP, accumulates during hypoxia (Saugstad, 1988). When subsequently oxidized during the recovery phase to xanthine and uric acid, highly reactive and toxic oxygen free radicals may be produced, temporarily overwhelming the scavenger systems. Intraneuronal calcium accumulation may lead to arachidonate release from membrane phospholipids, which when oxidized to prostaglandins or leukotrienes may impair local perfusion, thus aggravating the injury, and also produce further free radicals (Siesjo, 1981).

Delayed Cell Death

Post-insult excitotoxic activity and the resultant calcium influx (Siesjo, 1981; Choi, 1988) has been postulated as contributing to delayed neuronal death. This damage occurs in regions with a high density of glutaminergic projections (Wieloch, 1985) and may result from: excessive secretion of excitatory amino acids (Benveniste et al., 1984); failure of re-uptake (Silverstein et al., 1986a); greater sensitivity of inhibitory neurones to asphyxial insults (Sloper et al., 1980; Romijn et al., 1988); or their down-regulation (Lee et al., 1986). It has been suggested that post-asphyxic excitotoxic activity may be reflected in clinically apparent seizures (Siesjo, 1986) and that this may contribute to cell loss (Brown et al., 1979).

Endogenous Responses to Asphyxia

Not all insults lead to damage and endogenous protective responses include the release of a number of inhibitory neurotransmitters and neuromodulators which inhibit calcium flux and counteract the excitotoxins. For example, adenosine and some endogenous opiates are reported to be increased post-asphyxia (Lagercrantz et al., 1986; Dragunow and Faull, 1988; Hall and Pazara, 1988). Of concern is the current use of adenosine antagonists such as theophylline in apnoeic infants. This practice may exacerbate asphyxic brain damage. Also worrisome is the fact that glucocorticoid administration can increase hypoxic-ischaemic damage (Sapolsky, 1987). Thus, use of these in the fetus at risk or as anti-oedema agents in the asphyxiated neonate could worsen neurological outcome.

It is probable that the relative importance of these processes varies with the nature and severity of the insult, the cerebral structure concerned, age, and the metabolic status preceding, during, and after the insult. For example, hyperglycaemia often worsens neurological outcome but mild hypoglycaemia post-insult can improve outcome in rats (Voll and Auer, 1988; Voll et al., 1989). Nearly all experimental studies have been performed in healthy animals, whereas in the clinical situation asphyxial insults are often repeated or superimposed on pre-existing metabolic compromise. Recently it has been clearly demonstrated that neural maturation may be altered by intrauterine growth retardation (IUGR) (Cook et al., 1988) and that in the fetal guinea pig IUGR is associated with a greater sensitivity to asphyxia (Thordstein and Kjellmer, 1988). Similarly, severely growth-retarded term infants appear to be more sensitive to fetal hypoxaemia or birth asphyxia (Dijxhoorn et al., 1987). A number of early reports suggested that metabolic status might affect the global or regional sensitivity to asphyxia in the fetus (Myers et al., 1984) but definitive studies are lacking.

Asphyxic Insults: Experimental Approaches in the Fetus

We have used two different approaches to the induction of cerebral hypoxia-ischaemia in the fetal sheep; both result in similar patterns of neuronal loss. Severe asphyxia induced by either uterine artery occlusion or more than 20 minutes of transient cerebral ischaemia in the fetal sheep (119–126 days) leads to damage predominantly in the parasagittal cortex (Gunn et al., 1989b; Williams et al., 1990a). This pattern of damage is typical of ischaemic insults and has been observed after asphyxia in some term infants (Volpe and Hill, 1987) and in non-human primates (Brann and Myers, 1975). This distribution corresponds to the arterial end-fields in the border zones between the territories of the major cerebral arteries (anterior, middle, and posterior) (Brierley et al., 1969) and has been suggested as being a consequence of a period of impaired cerebral blood flow (Volpe and Hill, 1987). The relative sparing of midbrain and hindbrain structures such as the cerebellum when compared with the cortex, may reflect preferential perfusion of the residual flow to these structures as reported in fetal sheep and monkeys and in neonatal dogs, rats, and piglets during hypoxia-ischaemia or asphyxia (Behrman et al., 1970; Hernandez et al., 1979; Cavazzuti and Duff, 1982; Laptook et al., 1982; Ashwal et al., 1984; Vannucci et al., 1988). The developing brain is known to be particularly susceptible to excitotoxic injury (McDonald et al., 1988), perhaps as a consequence of delayed maturation of inhibitory processes (Michelson and Lothman, 1988) and thus this pattern of damage might also be a consequence of the distribution of glutamate receptors (Silverstein et al., 1987).

Potential Approaches to Therapeutic Intervention

It has only been with an improved understanding of the biochemical and neurophysiological processes leading to hypoxic-ischaemic neuronal death that there have been rational investigations into neuroprotective approaches. The wide range of mechanisms involved in neuronal injury suggests several approaches, which have been the subject of much experimental investigation, particularly in the mature animal. However, few studies (Silverstein et al., 1986b;

Gunn et al., 1989a) have considered the importance of developmenal state and the potential effects of intrauterine exposure. Most importantly the real problem is that these agents will be given to fetuses or neonates who are systemically unwell as opposed to animals in the pre-existing normal state. This concern has not yet been addressed directly.

Calcium Channel Antagonists

Calcium channel blockers, which might work either by improving cerebral blood flow or most likely via reducing non-specific voltage-dependent calcium entry (Beck et al., 1988) have been suggested as potential neuroprotective agents. We have extensively studied one such agent, flunarizine (Jansen, Beerse), which is unusual amongst calcium channel blockers in that it is lipid soluble and so crosses the placental and blood–brain barrier well (Holmes et al., 1984) with minimal cardiac depression.

Initial studies consisted of giving 30 mg/kg in divided doses 2 hours before hypoxia in the Levine infant rat model in which the rat with a unilateral carotid ligation is subject to inhalational asphyxia. Of the control animals, 50% had gross cerebral infarction on the ligated side, while in the flunarizine-treated animals the incidence of infarction was less than 4%. Detailed histological analysis confirmed that in all areas significant protection was achieved (Silverstein et al., 1986b; Gunn et al., 1989a).

In the fetal sheep the dosage of flunarizine appeared to be critical. If too much was given, systemic hypotension occurred. This could compromise the brain or cause fetal death (45 mg over 2 hours), particularly in growth-retarded chronically asphyxiated fetuses. Using a lower dose of 30 mg over 3 hours given as a fetal intravenous infusion, there was a significantly improved recovery as indicated by electrophysiological criteria at 72 hours post-insult ($p < 0.05$). The data indicate that flunarizine is indeed neuroprotective, at least to the cerebral cortex, when administered before an in utero insult. Given the very fast clearance of flunarizine from the fetal circulation the effect was probably during the insult and re-perfusion period.

Reactive or Re-perfusion Phase: Free Radical Scavengers

Free-radical scavengers (Abe et al., 1988) or drugs that control cerebral oedema (Sutherland et al., 1988) may have neuroprotective actions, at least in mature experimental animal models. Such agents may have a therapeutic role in the management of the asphyxiated neonate or fetus. For example, Thiringer et al. (1987) have demonstrated that immediate post-insult infusion of a mixture of free-radical scavengers, calcium-channel antagonists and anti-oedema agents improves the short-term neurological recovery (2 hours) after asphyxia in the newborn lamb. However, the long-term outcome was not assessed.

Prevention of Delayed Neuronal Death: The Use of Anticonvulsants

The next question which we have started to address is whether post-insult epileptiform activity contributes to neuronal loss. Given that in the majority of babies therapy will only be possible after identification of the insult, strategies that reduce delayed neuronal death will be particularly important.

Intense epileptiform activity leads to spreading depolarization in the neocortex (Hablitz and Heinemann, 1989), oedema and cell death in vitro (Watson et al., 1989). In adult rats epileptiform activity for more than 30 minutes can cause rapid neuronal death (Nevander et al., 1985; Ingvar et al., 1988), and the onset of post-ischaemic convulsions is closely coupled with the delayed death of cortical neurones (Smith et al., 1988). In clinical studies, early onset of post-asphyxial seizures and prolonged seizures are early predictors of which infants will die or have significant neurological sequelae (Mellits et al., 1982; Tudehope et al., 1988). Thus the hyperactivity of 6 ± 5 hours seen from 9 hours after 30 minutes of transient cerebral ischaemia in the fetal sheep may have contributed to neuronal loss (Williams et al., 1990a).

It has been suggested that epileptic damage occurs as a consequence of metabolic demands exceeding limited energy substrate availability in vulnerable neurones and not local hypoxia-ischaemia: so-called 'hypermetabolic' necrosis (Nevander et al., 1985; Auer et al., 1986). This damage is associated with local lactate accumulation (Kuhr and Korf, 1988). It is interesting to note that mild post-insult hypoglycaemia can improve outcome in an adult ischaemia rat preparation that shows post-ischaemic seizures (Voll and Auer, 1988). Thus post-asphyxic metabolic state may play an important role in determining outcome.

Impedance measurements can be used to assess intracellular oedema (Van Harreveld et al., 1971; Pelligrino et al., 1981). We have applied a robust four-electrode technique to measure parietal cortical oedema following cerebral ischaemia in the fetal sheep. These measurements show an acute, rapidly reversible oedema then a delayed secondary swelling during the period of low-frequency epileptiform activity, peaking at about 30 hours post-insult (Williams and Gluckman, 1989). This delayed oedema was persistent and associated with severe cortical neuronal loss (laminar necrosis) at 3 days post ischaemia (Williams and Gluckman, 1989). Similarly, adult rats show a secondary oedema associated with the onset of post-ischaemic convulsions (Warner et al., 1987). Intracranial pressure measurements in severely asphyxiated infants show a comparable time course of delayed oedema peaking at about 48 hours, which also is associated with poor neurological outcome (Lupton et al., 1988).

Studies in both adult and neonatal animal preparations indicate that secondary oedema is closely coupled with cell death and probably is a consequence rather than a cause of necrosis (Rice et al., 1981; Petito et al., 1982; Ames and Nesbett, 1983; Kumar et al., 1987; Mujsce et al., 1987). Thus the secondary swelling during and persisting after the epileptiform activity suggests that this epileptiform activity is closely coupled with delayed cell death.

The concept of post-asphyxial therapeutic intervention is not new: barbiturates have been repeatedly tried but have not shown any consistent benefit either experimentally or in humans (Goldberg et al., 1986; Trauner, 1986). Commonly used anticonvulsants (phenobarbitone, paraldehyde, phenytoin, and diazepam) are often ineffective at treating post-asphyxic seizures in neonates (Eyre and Wilkinson, 1986; Connell et al., 1989). In addition even when the clinical seizures are abolished by phenobarbital, epileptiform activity may persist (Mizrahi, 1987). Status epilepticus may involve a failure of GABA-ergic inhibition (Gloor, 1989); thus GABA agonists such as barbiturates are not likely to be effective against these seizures. Further the origin of post-asphyxial seizures is likely to result from activity of the excitatory amino acids. Thus therapeutic intervention is more likely to be successful if the activity of these transmitters is reduced.

We have begun studies of post-insult administration of a potent anticonvulsant and NMDA receptor antagonist, MK-801, to resolve the role of post-asphyxic epileptiform activity. Doses of MK-801 between 0.5 and 2 mg given to the sheep fetus are effective in treating status epilepticus induced by central administered penicillin, while barbiturates, which are functionally GABA-ergic agonists, are not (Gunn et al., 1988).

The proto-oncogene c-*fos* has been suggested as being involved in the processes of neuronal repair or death after seizures or ischaemia. In the Levine infant rat model c-*fos* induction does not occur in the infarcted region of the ligated hemisphere, probably due to early neuronal failure. However, induction is very marked on the non-ligated side where there is no neuronal loss. Both this contralateral induction and the convulsions were abolished by the anticonvulsant, MK-801 (Gunn et al., 1990). Interestingly, c-*fos* protein induction did appear on the ligated side after MK-801 pretreatment, consistent with its reported neuroprotective effects (McDonald et al., 1987; Hattori et al., 1989), but doses > 0.5 mg/kg were associated with increased mortality ($p < 0.001$). Similarly, in our studies in fetal sheep, MK-801 administration prior to the insult completely abolished post-ischaemic seizures, but in higher doses was associated with increased fetal mortality.

Although post-asphyxial seizure activity is probably harmful, careful assessment of the functional benefits of anticonvulsants is needed. A case in point is chronic exposure to the GABA-ergic anticonvulsant, diazepam, after unilateral cortical damage. Evidence suggests that this anticonvulsant can retard functional recovery (Brailowsky et al., Schallert et al., 1986). In contrast, administration of a GABA-ergic antagonist after 1 day post-insult appears to accelerate functional recovery (Hernandez and Schallert, 1988). This suggests that excessive use of some anticonvulsants may be harmful. Indeed Hernandez and Schallert (1988) have suggested that partial, rather than complete, suppression of seizures may favourably affect functional recovery. The relationship between synaptic activity growth and plasticity is increasingly recognized in developmental biology and presumably this relationship is also important in the functional repair and recovery processes.

Identification of an Asphyxic Insult

Although a period of severe asphyxia can clearly lead to hypoxic-ischaemic encephalopathy (Freeman, 1985; Volpe and Hill, 1987), many asphyxiated infants rapidly recover without neurological abnormalities. The severity of a perinatal asphyxic insult is difficult to assess (Dijxhoorn et al., 1986). Commonly used indices of asphyxia at birth, such as low Apgar score, acidaemia, and the presence of amniotic meconium, have little value by themselves in predicting neurological outcome (Dijxhoorn et al., 1986; Marrin and Paes, 1988; Dennis et al., 1989). Similarly, some fetal sheep can withstand 30–60 minutes of asphyxia ($CaO_2 = 1.0$ mM) and rapidly recover cortical function with little or no neuronal loss (Parer et al., 1989). However, in others this asphyxia can lead to brain damage (Gunn et al., 1989b). Improved early identification of the asphyxiated infants likely to develop brain damage may enable appropriate recovery strategies to be applied to reduce the damage initiated by severe asphyxia.

The relationship between severity of the insult and subsequent pathogenesis was investigated in the fetal sheep ischaemia model (119–126 days) (Williams et al., 1990b). Parietal EEG activity was continuously analysed with real-time spectral intensity analysis (Williams and Gluckman, 1990) and histological outcome was assessed at 3 days post-ischaemia. Two patterns of response were found. Following a mild insult (10 minutes of ischaemia) the parietal EEG showed gradual recovery toward normal activity with mild neuronal loss. Severe insults (more than 20 minutes of ischaemia) showed 8 ± 2 hours of suppressed EEG followed by an increase in low-frequency activity then gradual loss of intensity seen with severe neuronal death (laminar necrosis) in the underlying parasagittal cortex at 3 days post-ischaemia. After 30 minutes of ischaemia there was a period of hyperactivity that peaked at 9 ± 1 hours ($p < 0.005$) with intensity 7 ± 3 dB greater than control levels (Williams et al., 1990b). This increased low-frequency activity was apparent as spike-wave or epileptiform activity on the raw EEG and occurred with both tonic and clonic convulsions (Williams et al., 1990a). The sequence of initial suppression, then delayed seizures followed by loss of activity seen with cortical damage, shows similarities to the progression of some asphyxiated term infants (Volpe and Hill, 1987), near miss

SIDs infants (Aubourg et al., 1985; Constantinou et al., 1989) and adults following hypoxic-ischaemic insults (Madison and Niedermeyer, 1970; Snyder et al., 1980a, 1980b).

Two parietal electrophysiological criteria were both found to predict severe neuronal loss in the underlying cortex at 3 days following a hypoxic-ischaemic insult: suppression for more than 5 hours followed by a period of increased low-frequency EEG activity with a median frequency less than 8 Hz (Williams et al., 1990b).

Furthermore, both the loss of EEG intensity and secondary cortical oedema at 3 days post-insult were associated with severe parasagittal laminar necrosis (Williams and Gluckman, 1989; Williams et al., 1990b). Thus continuous EEG monitoring and analysis immediately post-asphyxia may facilitate identification of infants likely to develop neurological deficits. Furthermore, this will improve detection of potentially damaging periods of epileptiform activity (Eyre et al., 1983; Connell et al., 1989) in asphyxiated infants and facilitate the assessment of the effectiveness of anticonvulsant treatment (Eyre et al., 1983).

Conclusions

Together the studies show that therapeutic intervention both before and after asyphyxia is possible by manipulation of a number of processes. Each particular approach reflects only a few facets of the complex spectrum of mechanisms involved in the generation of perinatal encephalopathy. However, while early experimental data are promising it is clear that application to the clinical situation must proceed with caution. Virtually all studies have been performed in animals with no pre-existing metabolic compromise. Agents such as NMDA receptor antagonists and calcium channel blockers may well have side-effects which hinder their application in the compromised fetus or neonate. Indeed, limited data with both flunarizine and MK-801 suggest caution is warranted. Flunarizine at high doses may interfere with uterine and fetal cardiovascular status (Harake et al., 1987). Consequently, a still wider range of experimental approaches in large animal preparations and therapeutic methodologies clearly must be tested to establish their efficacy and safety before clinical trials can be considered.

Much remains to be learned about the precise pathophysiology of fetal asphyxia. The delayed epileptiform activity seen with a rise in cerebral oedema suggests that this hyperactivity may contribute to delayed cell death and indicates a possible window of opportunity for therapeutic intervention. The application of improved techniques of continuous EEG monitoring to asphyxiated infants should enable development of more effective criteria for rapid prediction of neurological outcome and improve detection of potentially damaging periods of epileptiform activity in asphyxiated infants.

Acknowledgements

These studies were supported by grants from the Medical Research Council of New Zealand, the Neurological Foundation of New Zealand, and the National Children's Health Research Foundation.

References

Abe K, Yuki S, Kogure K (1988) Strong attenuation of ischemic and postischemic brain edema in rats by a novel free radical scavenger. Stroke 19: 480–485.

Ames A and Nesbett F (1983) Pathophysiology of ischemic cell death: II. Changes in plasma membrane permeability and cell volume. Stroke 14: 227–233.

Ashwal S, Dale P, Longo L (1984) Regional cerebral blood flow: studies in the fetal lamb during hypoxia, hypercapnia, acidosis, and hypotension. Pediatr Res 18: 1309–1984.

Aubourg P, Dulac O, Plouin P, Diebler C (1985) Infantile status epilepticus as a complication of 'Near-miss' sudden infant death. Dev Med Child Neurol 27: 40–48.

Auer R, Ingvar M, Nevander G, Olsson Y, Siesjo B (1986) Early axonal lesion and preserved microvasculature in epilepsy-induced hypermetabolic necrosis of the substantia nigra. Acta Neuropathol (Berl) 71: 207–215.

Beck T, Nuglisch J, Sauer D, Bielenberg B, Mennel H, Rossberg C, Kreglstein J (1988) Effects of flunarizine on postischemic blood flow, energy metabolism and neuronal damage in the rat brain. Eur J Pharmacol 158: 271–274.

Behrman R, Lees M, Peterson E, De Lannoy C, Seeds A (1970) Distribution of the circulation in the normal and asphyxiated fetal primate. Am J Obstet Gynec 108: 956–969.

Bejar R, Wozniak P, Allard M, Bernirschke K, Baucher Y, Coen R, Berry C, Schragg P, Villegas I, Resnik R (1988) Antenatal origin of neurologic damage in newborn infants. Am J Obstet Gynecol 159: 357–363.

Beneveniste H, Drejer J, Schousboe A, Diemer H (1984) Elevation of the extracellular concentration of glutamate and aspartate in rat hippocampus during transient brain ischemia monitored by intracerebral microdialysis. J Neurochem 43: 1369–1374.

Brailowsky S, Knight R, Blood K, Scabini D (1986) GABA-induced potentiation of cortical hemiplegia. Brain Res 362: 322–330.

Brann A and Myers R (1975) Central nervous system findings in the newborn monkey following severe in utero partial asphyxia. Neurol 25: 327–338.

Brierley J, Brown A, Excell B, Meldrum B (1969) Brain damage in the Rhesus monkey from profound arterial hypotension. Brain Res 13: 68–100.

Brown A, Levy E, Kublik M (1979) Selective chromatolysis of neurons in the gerbil brain: a possible consequence of 'epileptic' activity produced by common carotid artery occlusion. Ann Neurol 5: 127–138.

Cavazzuti M and Duffy T (1982) Regulation of local cerebral blood flow in normal and hypoxic newborn dogs. Ann Neurol 11: 247–257.

Choi D (1988) Calcium mediated neurotoxicity: relationship to specific channel types and role in ischemic damage. TINS 11: 465–469.

Connell J, Oozeer R, De Vries L, Dubowitz L, Dubowitz V (1989) Clinical and EEG response to anticonvulsants in neonatal seizures. Arch Dis Child 64: 459–464.

Constantinou J, Gillis J, Ouvrier R, Rahilly P (1989) Hypoxic-ischemic encephalopathy after near miss sudden infant death syndrome. Arch Dis Child 64: 703–708.

Cook C, Gluckman P, Williams C, Bennet L (1988) Precocial neural function in the growth retarded fetal lamb. Ped Res 24: 600–605.

Dean R (1987) Some critical membrane events during mammalian cell death. In: Perspectives on Mammalian Cell Death (Ed: Potten CS), pp. 18–38. Oxford Science Publications, New York.

Dennis J, Johnson A, Mutch L, Yudkin P, Johnson P (1989) Acid-base status at birth and neurodevelopmental outcome at four and one-half years. Am J Obstet Gynecol 171: 213–220.

Dijxhoorn M, Visser G, Fidler V, Touwen B, Huisjes H (1986) Apgar score, meconium and acidaemia at birth in relation to neonatal neurological morbidity. Br J Obstet Gynaecol 93: 217–222.

Dijxhoorn M, Visser G, Touwen B, Huisjes H (1987) Apgar score, meconium and acidemia at birth in small-for-gestational age infants born at term, and their relation to neonatal neurological morbidity. Br J Obstet Gynaecol 94: 873–879.

Dragunow M and Faull R (1988) Neuroprotective effects of adenosine. TIPS 9: 193–194.

Eyre J and Wilkinson A (1986) Thiopentone induced coma after severe birth asphyxia. Arch Dis Child 61: 1084–1089.

Eyre J, Oozeer R, Wilkinson A (1983) Diagnosis of neonatal seizure by continuous recording and rapid analysis of the electroencephalogram. Arch Dis Child 58: 785–790.

Freeman J (Ed) (1985) Prenatal and Perinatal Factors Associated with Brain Disorders. NIH Pub 85-1149.

Gloor P (1989) Epilepsy: relationships between electrophysiology and intracellular mechanisms involving second messengers and gene expression. Le Canadien J Neurol Sci 16: 8–21.

Goldberg R, Moscosos P, Bloom F, Curless R, Burke B, Bancalari F (1986) Use of barbiturate therapy in severe perinatal asphyxia: a randomized controlled trial. J Pediatr 109(5): 851–856.

Gunn A, Bennet L, Williams C, Gluckman P (1988) The behavioral and anticonvulsant effects of MK-801, an amino acid antagonist, in the ovine fetus and ewe. Proc Liggins Symp, Rotorua, p. 19 (abstr).

Gunn A, Mydlar T, Bennet L, Faull R, Gorter S, Cook C, Johnston B, Gluckman P (1989a) The neuroprotective actions of a calcium channel antagonist, flunarizine, in the infant rat. Ped Res 25: 573–576.

Gunn A, Parer J, Mallard C, Gluckman P (1989b) Cerebral histological damage following acute reduction of uterine blood flow in the fetal sheep. Proc Soc Study Fetal Phys, Reading, p. C1 (abstr).

Gunn A, Dragunow M, Faull R, Gluckman P (1990) Hypoxia-ischemia and seizures have opposed effects on neuronal c-fos protein levels in the infant rat. Brain Res (in press).

Hablitz J and Heinemann U (1989) Alterations in the microenvironment during spreading depression associated with epileptiform activity in the immature cortex. Dev Brain Res 46: 243–252.

Hall E and Pazara K (1988) Quantitative analysis of effects of K-opioid agonists on postischemic hippocampal CA1 neuronal necrosis in gerbils. Stroke 19: 1008–1012.

Harake B, Gilbert R, Ashwal S, Power G (1987) Nifedipine: effects on fetal and maternal hemodynamics in pregnant sheep. Am J Obstet Gynecol 157: 1003–1008.

Hattori H, Morin A, Schwartz P, Fujikawa D, Wasterlain C (1989) Posthypoxic treatment with MK-801 reduces hypoxic-ischemic damage in the neonatal rat. Neurology 39: 713–718.

Hernandez M, Hawkins R, Brennan R, Vannucci R, Helm B, Bowman G (1979) Redistribution of regional cerebral blood flow during neonatal asphyxia. Acta Neurol Scand 60(suppl 71): 288–289.

Hernandez T and Schallert T (1988) Seizures and recovery from brain damage. Exp Neurol 102: 318–324.

Hill A and Volpe J (1982) Hypoxic-ischaemic brain injury in the newborn. Seminars in Perinatology 6(1): 25–41.

Holmes B, Brogdenm R, Heel R, Speight T, Avery G (1984) Flunarizine: a review of its pharmacodynamic and pharmacokinetic properties and therapeutic use. Drugs 27: 6–44.

Ingvar M, Morgan P, Auer R (1988) The nature and timing of excitotoxic neuronal necrosis in the cerebral cortex, hippocampus and thalamus due to flurothyl-induced status epilepticus. Acta Neuropathol (Berl) 75: 362–369.

Kirino T (1982) Delayed neuronal death in the gerbil hippocampus following ischemia. Brain Res 239: 57–69.

Kuhr W and Korf J (1988) N-methyl-D-aspartate involvement in lactate production following ischemia or convulsion in rats. Euro J Pharmac 155: 145–149.

Kumar K, Goosmann M, Krause G, Nayini N, Estrada R, Hoehner T, White B, Koestner A (1987) Neuropathol (Berl) 73: 393–399.

Lagercrantz H, Fredholm BB, Irestedt L, Runold M, Sollevi A (1986) Adenosine—a neuromodulatory released during asphyxia and a mediator of some hypoxic effects in the newborn? Cardiovascular Resp Physiol Fetus and Neonate 133: 153–160.

Laptook A, Stonestreet B, Oh W (1982) The effects of different rates of plasmanate infusions upon brain blood flow after asphyxia and hypotension in newborn piglets. J Pediatr 100(5): 791–796.

Lee K, Tetzlaff W, Kreutzberg G (1986) Rapid down regulation of hippocampal adenosine receptors following brief anoxia. Brain Res 360: 155–158.

Low J, Robertson D, Simpson L (1989) Temporal relationships of neuropathologic conditions caused by perinatal asphyxia. Am J Obstet Gynecol 160: 608–614.

Lupton B, Hill A, Roland E, Whitfield M, Flodmark O (1988) Brain swelling in the asphyxiated term newborn: pathogenesis and outcome. Pediatrics 82: 139–146.

Madison D and Niedermeyer E (1970) Epileptic seizures resulting from acute cerebral anoxia. Journal of Neurology, Neurosurgery and Psychiatry. 33: 381–386.

Marrin M and Paes B (1988) Does the Apgar score have diagnostic value? Obstet Gynecol 72: 120–123.

McDonald J, Silverstein F, Johnston M (1987) MK-801 protects the neonatal brain from hypoxic-ischemic damage. European Journal of Pharmacology 140: 359–361.

McDonald J, Silverstein F, Johnston M (1988) Neurotoxicity of N-methyl-D-aspartate is markedly enhanced in developing rat central nervous system. Brain Res 459: 200–203.

Mellits E, Holden K, Freeman J (1982) Neonatal seizures II. A multivariate analysis of factors associated with outcome. Pediatrics 70: 177–185.

Michelson H and Lothman E (1988) An in vivo electrophysiological study of the ontogeny of excitatory and inhibitory processes in the rat hippocampus. Dev Brain Res 47: 113–122.

Mizrahi E (1987) Neonatal seizures: problems in diagnosis and classification. Epilepsia 28(S1): S46–S55.

Mujsce D, Boyer M, Vannucci R (1987) CBF and brain edema in perinatal cerebral hypoxia-ischemia. Pediatr Res 21: 494A.

Mulligan J, Painter M, O'Donoghue P (1980) Neonatal asphyxia II. Neonatal mortality and long-term sequelae. J Pediatr 96: 903.

Myers R, DeCourten-Myers GM, Wagner KR (1984) Effect of hypoxia on fetal brain.

In: Fetal Physiology and Medicine, 2nd edn (Eds: Beard RW and Nathanielsz PW), pp. 419–458. Marcel Dekker: New York.

Nevander G, Ingvar M, Auer R, Siesjo B (1985) Status epilepticus in well-oxygenated rats causes neuronal necrosis. Ann Neurol 18: 281–290.

Parer J, Williams C, Gunn A, Gluckman P (1989) Electrocorticographic changes during acute severe uterine blood flow reduction in fetal sheep. Proc Soc Gyn Invest.

Pelligrino D, Almquist L, Siesjo B (1981) Effects of insulin-induced hypoglycemia on intracellular pH and impedance in the cerebral cortex of the rat. Brain Res 221: 129–147.

Petito C, Pulsinelli W, Jacobson G, Plum F (1982) Edema and vascular permeability in cerebral ischemia: comparison between ischemic neuronal damage and infarction. J Neuropathol Exp Neurol 41(4): 423–436.

Pulsinelli W, Brierley J, Plum F (1982) Temporal profile of neuronal damage in a model of transient forebrain ischemia. Ann Neurol 11: 491–498.

Rice J, Vannucci R, Brierley J (1981) The influence of immaturity on hypoxic-ischemic brain damage in the rat. Ann Neurol 9: 131–141.

Robertson C, Finer N, Grace M (1989) School performance of survivors of neonatal encephalopathy associated with birth asphyxia at term. J Pediatr 114: 753–760.

Romijn H, Ruijter J, Wolters P (1988) Hypoxia preferentially destroys GABAergic neurons in developing rat neocortex explants in culture. Exp Neurol 100: 332–340.

Rothman S and Olney J (1987) Excitotoxicity and the NMDA receptor. TINS 10: 299–302.

Sapolsky R (1987) Glucocorticoids and hippocampal damage. TINS 10(9): 346–349.

Saugstad O (1988) Hypoxanthine as an indicator of hypoxia: its role in health and disease through free radical production. Ped Res 23: 143–150

Schallert T, Hernandez T, Barth T (1986) Recovery of function after brain damage: severe and chronic disruption by diazepam. Brain Res 379: 104–11.

Siesjo B (1981) Cell damage in the brain: a speculative synthesis. J Cereb Blood Flow Metab 1: 155–185.

Siesjo B (1986) Cellular calcium metabolism, seizures and ischemia. Mayo Clin Proc 61: 299–302.

Silverstein F, Buchanan K, Johnston M (1986a) Perinatal hypoxia-ischaemia disrupts striatal high-affinity (3H)-glutamate uptake into synaptosomes. J Neurochem 47: 1614–1619.

Silverstein F, Buchanan K, Hudson C, Johnston M (1986b) Flunarizine limits hypoxic-ischaemia induced morphologic injury in immature rat brain. Stroke 17: 477–482.

Silverstein F, Torke L, Barks J, Johnston M (1987) Hypoxia-ischemia produces focal disruption of glutamate receptors in developing brain. Dev Brain Res 34: 33–39.

Sloper J, Johnson P, Powell T (1980) Selective degeneration of interneurons in the motor cortex of infant monkeys following controlled hypoxia: a possible cause of epilepsy. Brain Res 198: 204–209.

Smith M, Kalimo H, Warner D, Siesjo B (1988) Morphological lesions in the brain preceding the development of postischemic seizures. Acta Neuropathol 76: 253–264.

Snyder B, Houser W, Loewenson R, Leppik I, Ramirez Lassepas M, Gumnit R (1980a) Neurologic prognosis after cardiopulmonary arrest. III: Seizure activity. Neurology 30: 1292–1297.

Snyder B, Loewenson R, Gumnit R, Houser W, Leppik I, Ramirez Lassepas M (1980b) Neurologic prognosis after cardiopulmonary arrest. II: Level of consciousness. Neurology 30: 52–58.

Steenbergen C and Jennings R (1984) Relationship between lysophospholipid accumulation and plasma membrane injury during total in vitro ischemia in dog heart. J Mol Cell Cardiol 16: 605–621.

Sutherland G, Lesiuk H, Bose R, Sima A (1988) Effect of mannitol, nimodipine and indomethacin singly or in combination on cerebral ischemia in rats. Stroke 19: 571–578.

Thiringer K, Hrbek Z, Karlsson K, Rosen K, Kjellmer I (1987) Postasphyxial cerebral survival in newborn sheep after treatment with oxygen free radical scavengers and a calcium channel antagonist. Pediatr Res 22: 62–67.

Thordstein M and Kjellmer I (1988) Cerebral tolerance of hypoxia in growth retarded and appropriately grown newborn guinea pigs. Pediatr Res 24: 633–638.

Trauner D (1986) Barbiturate therapy in acute brain injury. J Pediatr 109: 742–746.

Tudehope D, Harris A, Hawes D, Hayes M (1988) Clinical spectrum and outcome of neonatal convulsions. Aust Paediatr J 24: 249–253.

Uematsu D, Greenberg J, Reivich M, Karp A (1988) In vivo measurement of cytosolic free calcium during cerebral ischaemia and reperfusion. Ann Neurol 24: 420–428.

Van der Vusse G, Van Bilsen M, Reneman R (1989) Is phospholipid degradation a critical event in ischemia and reperfusion-induced damage. NIPS 4: 49–53.

Van Harreveld A, Dafny N, Khattab F (1971) Effects of calcium on the electrical resistance and the extracellular space of cerebral cortex. Exp Neurol 31: 358–367.

Vannucci R, Lyons D, Vasta F (1988) Regional cerebral blood flow during hypoxia-ischemia in immature rats. Stroke 19: 245–250.

Voll C and Auer R (1988) The effect of postischemic blood glucose levels on ischemic brain damage in the rat. Ann Neurol 24: 638–646.

Voll C, Whishaw I, Auer R (1989) Postischemic insulin reduces spatial learning deficit following transient forebrain ischemia in rats. Stroke 20: 646–651.

Volpe J and Pasernak J (1977) Parasagittal cerebral injury in neonatal hypoxic-ischemic injury. J Pediatr 91: 472–476.

Volpe J and Hill A (1987) Neurologic disorders. In: Neonatology and Management of the Newborn 3rd edn (Ed: Avery G), pp. 1073–1132. JB Lippincott, Philadelphia.

Warner D, Smith M, Siesjo B (1987) Ischemia in normo- and hyperglycemic rats: effects on brain water and electrolytes. Stroke 18: 464–471.

Watson G, Rader R, Lanthorn T (1989) Epileptiform activity in vitro can produce long-term synaptic failure and persistent neuronal depolarisation. Brain Res 498: 81–88.

Wieloch T (1985) Neurochemical correlates to selective neuronal vulnerability. Progr Br Res 63: 69–85.

Williams C and Gluckman P (1989) Delayed edema with hypoxic-ischemic encephalopathy in the fetal sheep. Proc Satellite Symposium Recovery from Brain Damage IUPS p. 34.

Williams C and Gluckman P (1990) Real-time spectral intensity analysis of the EEG on a microcomputer. J Neurosci Meth 32: 9–13.

Williams C, Gunn A, Gluckman P, Synek B (1990a) Delayed seizures occurring with hypoxic-ischemic encephalopathy in the fetal sheep. Pediatr Res 27(6): 561–565.

Williams C, Gunn A, Mallard C, Gluckman P (1990b) The pathogenesis of HIE following different durations of cerebral ischemia in the fetal sheep. J Clin Invest (submitted).

Discussion

In reply to questions about examination of the brains, Dr Williams said that the sheep were killed 72 hours after the episode of ischaemia, fixed by perfusion with 10% formalin in situ, serially sectioned and the sections stained with acid fuchsin. Ischaemia was caused by tying of the vertebral-carotid arterial anastomoses, and by occluding the carotid arteries by occlusion cuffs, after 3 days recovery from surgical preparation, which was done under anaesthesia. Ischaemia was maintained for 10 or 40 minutes. There may, of course, have been continued anastomotic perfusion of parts of the brainstem through the circle of Willis. He had used total ischaemia, rather than partial asphyxia or hypoxia, because the latter were more difficult to standardize. John Patrick pointed out that ischaemia with recovery was a classic way to induce a reperfusion injury. Williams could not answer Thornburg's enquiry as to what protection, if any, is afforded by an earlier gestational age, or in a mature fetus as compared with a newborn lamb, because the observations had only been carried out at one gestational age. In reply to a further question from Thornburg about the relative sensitivity to ischaemia of different areas of the brain, it appeared that no exact relationship had been established with the relative blood flows (per unit of tissue) as measured by Ashwal et al. (1980), for example.

Ellendorf asked whether pH, pO_2 or pCO_2 had been measured locally in the brain. There might be interesting differences with gestational age and/or in different areas. Williams described the difficulty of such measurements in chronic fetal lamb preparations; he thought it would be useful to make local measurements of lactate and glutamate if that were possible.

Patrick recalled that Peter Gluckman, in a meeting in June 1989 in Oxford, had reported preliminary results that glutaminergic blockers were effective at preventing seizures but not lesions. Williams confirmed that such blockers were effective anticonvulsants; he was not so sure as to their efficacy otherwise.

Possible Effects of Gestational Age

Hanson was curious as to when the physiological systems develop which afford some degree of natural protection from ischaemic damage. He wondered why they were so much less effective in the adult; what possible advantage was there in abandoning them? The subsequent discussion revealed that there was no precise information as to developmental changes in resistance to ischaemia in sheep. The fetus was allegedly more likely to be exposed to asphyxia, though apnoeic attacks were common in some infants postnatally. There was a great development of the brain after birth, the ratio of neurones to glia may change, and there was possibly adaptation to a higher pO_2 though this did not imply much increase in O_2 supply or tissue pO_2. Patrick pointed out that, in the mouse and rat, superoxide dismutase develops after birth, while Thornburg raised the possibility that the young fetus was less capable of generating free radicals in the brain during ischaemia and reperfusion (Vlessis and Mela-Riker, 1989).

Brain Damage and Birth Asphyxia

Redman discussed the relation between birth asphyxia and brain damage. When babies were found to have brain damage the obstetrician is usually blamed and financial damages are awarded accordingly. But he did not know what the truth was, i.e. whether there was a causal connection in all or any such cases. Scientists and obstetricians try to learn from animal models, such as that which Williams described, but these models may not correspond to what happens in the human infant perinatally. What does birth asphyxia mean and how does it relate to the forms of cerebral injury which occur?

Patrick had studied fetal lambs at 125–130 days gestation, exposed to 8 hours severe hypoxia with 3 days recovery (Richardson et al., 1989). Two of seven such lambs had periodic seizures lasting 2–3 minutes and, although apparently wholly recovered as shown by electrocortical activity, measurements of heart rate, fetal breathing, and rapid eye movements, there was preliminary evidence of laminar necrosis of the cerebral cortex. This was disturbing because the obstetrician might have no clinical evidence to guide him other than the presence of seizures, which were evident in only two of seven damaged fetuses.

Redman said that in clinical practice asphyxia was regarded as central nervous dysfunction with evidence of gross respiratory deprivation, defined as a low Apgar score at delivery (≤ 3 at 1 minute) combined with severe metabolic acidaemia. There is a gradation of acidaemia with increasing hypoxaemia. If brain depression is secondary then we should seek numerical standards of acidaemia to assess the degree of brain dysfunction. Visser wished to maintain a clear differentiation between a low Apgar score and metabolic acidaemia. Data from Groningen had shown that term fetuses with a *low Apgar score and normal blood gas values* at delivery were at higher risk of neurological morbidity than ones with 'classical asphyxia' (i.e. with a low pH, low base excess and low Apgar score; Dijxhoorn et al., 1986). When an infant does not soon start breathing after birth, one should ask the question whether this is due to drugs given to the mother, to gross metabolic acidaemia, to a low p_aO_2 or to pre-existing brain dysfunction. A low Apgar score might be more a marker of defective reactions as a result of other insults, rather than an index of hypoxaemia (see, for example, the follow-up of the 1970 British Birth Survey; Peters et al., 1984). He did not know how much O_2 lack was required to cause brain dysfunction clinically.

Pardi remarked that you can observe brain damage with normal blood gas values at delivery, so why should (classical) asphyxia be causally related? [There is good evidence from experiments on rhesus monkeys that asphyxia, prolonged for more than 10 minutes, by cord occlusion with prevention of breathing, induces brain damage; this can be prevented by infusion of alkali (Adamsons et al., 1963; Dawes et al., 1964), but this only shows that such a relationship is possible]. Visser thought that the effects of O_2 lack and acidaemia on brain function were dependent on gestational age. *At term* he and his colleagues could find no relation between umbilical arterial or venous pH at birth and neonatal neurological outcome. Furthermore, in 60 infants delivered with an umbilical arterial pH < 7.00, long-term outcome was the same as in a control group (Aarnoudse et al., 1985). Abnormal neurological outcome was concentrated in a group with a normal pH at delivery *and* a normal or low Apgar score. Dawes asked whether he was prepared to speculate as to the cause of the neurological abnormality in the latter group. Visser thought there were likely to be two causes: first, genetic or disorders during early development, since many infants found to be abnormal neurologically have minor morphological anomalies elsewhere (16–30%); second, there might also be transient antenatal cardiovascular events, for example associated with placental infarction, temporary cord occlusion, or prolonged pre-labour uterine contractions. In some reports a sudden cessation of fetal movements has been described, accompanied by a flat FHR pattern (gross attenuation of FHR variation); when labour was induced 1–2 days later the blood gas values on delivery during labour and at birth were normal.

Based on the course of the CT scan changes it was likely in one case that the 'hypoxic' insult had occurred some days before the onset of labour (Fricker et al., 1983). Recent literature indicated that central nervous system injuries occurring prior to the labour process are not rare (Barth, 1984; Sims et al., 1984; Paul et al., 1986; Mann, 1986). The causes include respiratory and circulatory accidents to the mother, abdominal trauma during pregnancy, twin pregnancy with a macerated co-twin, arterial occlusion of fetal cerebral vessels, placental insufficiency, and infections (Barth, 1984; Sims et al., 1985). At post-mortem, cerebral haemorrhage, gliosis, or porencephaly are found. Porencephaly may also be the result of genetic disease (Barth, 1984). Until now many of the surviving infants with such injuries have probably been left with 'unexplained' neurological handicaps, or handicaps thought to be due to the labour process. Antepartum FHR monitoring and prenatal ultrasound examinations might identify these cases and distinguish them from abnormalities of the nervous system acquired during and after birth.

Mandruzzato thought that it was not possible to give an unambiguous answer as to the cause of neurological abnormalities, first observed postnatally in fetuses whose perinatal progress had otherwise been normal. While obstetricians had been taught to believe that the quality of care was most important, in high-risk cases, especially with strict control, there was still insufficient information. Visser agreed that clinically the indicators of brain dysfunction, antenatally or in labour, were still poor.

Brain Damage, the Cerebral Circulation and Preceding Events

Pardi enquired whether evidence was available of the quality of neurological development in human fetuses in which there had been a large decrease of the pulsatility index (PI) in the cerebral circulation. Mandruzzato replied that he had found no evidence of neurological damage in infants in which the carotid arterial PI had decreased more than 2 SD below the mean value, appropriate for gestational age. Visser pointed out that most neurological abnormalities occurred in term fetuses, whose weight was appropriate for their age and sex; Pardi's question and Mandruzzato's reply were related to growth-retarded infants delivered prematurely.

Patrick said that evidence had been published (Low et al., 1989) of 17 autopsies on newborn infants in which the origin of the brain damage present must have been due to antepartum events; a considerable length of time—several days was required for the development of such lesions. In newborn infants CAT scans on the day of delivery also had shown, not uncommonly, the presence of such lesions. Dawes asked whether such antepartum events could explain some, or all, of the neurological sequelae hitherto attributed to birth asphyxia. Visser thought that the contribution of birth asphyxia itself was small, but did not give an estimate of the incidence where it either did or might have contributed in the second or third trimester.

Mandruzzato made the point that until 15 years ago perinatal mortality was much higher. It began to fall with the introduction of FHR monitoring in labour on selected high-risk cases. Visser was concerned about the relation between figures for perinatal mortality and morbidity. In the south of Sweden (Hagberg et al., 1984) perinatal mortality was still falling, but morbidity (including cerebral palsy), after an initial fall, had been rising steadily for 10 years in all birthweights. The obstetrician and the neonatologist, with improved intensive care, could ensure that relatively more infants survived, but there seemed to be a rise in the incidence of brain damage. Pardi agreed that prediction of fetal distress had improved, so that there were fewer fetal deaths in labour.

Dawes commented that if indeed 90% of all brain damage had occurred well before birth, that might alter Dr Williams' strategy. Was it possible to design observations which would help the obstetrician discover how and when brain damage occurs near term, for genetic reasons or otherwise? Cardiologists had discovered a great deal by 24-hour monitoring. A few obstetricians had looked at the fetus for up to 1–2 hours at a time, but rarely longer. Perhaps some longer records could be made, if prolonged ultrasound exposure or abdominal ECG recordings could be now regarded as safe.

References

Aarnoudse JG, Yspeert-Gerards, Touwen et al. (1985) International Workshop on Developmental Neurology of Fetus and Preterm Infant, Groningen, Holland.
Adamsons K, Behrman R, Dawes GS et al. (1963) J Physiol 169: 679–689.
Ashwall S, Majcher JS, Vain N et al. (1980) Ped Res 14: 1104–1110.
Barth PG (1984) Clin Neurol Neurosurg 86: 65–75.

Dawes GS, Hibbard E, Windle WF (1964) J Pediat 65: 801–806.

Dijxhoorn MJ, Visser GHA, Fidler et al. (1986) Br J Obstet Gynaecol 93: 217–222.

Fricker HS, Sauter M, Buchs B (1983) Ztsch für Geburtsh Perinatol 187: 50–53.

Hagberg B, Hagberg G, Olow I (1984) Acta Paediat Scand 73: 433–440.

Low JA, Robertson DH, Simpson LL (1989) Am J Obstet Gynecol 160: 608–614.

Mann LI (1986) Am J Obstet Gynecol 155: 6–10.

Paul RH, Yonekura ML, Cantrell CJ et al. (1986) Am J Obstet Gynecol 154: 1187–1190.

Peters TJ, Golding J, Lawrence DJ et al. (1984) Early Hum Dev 9: 225–240.

Richardson BS, Rurak D, Patrick J et al. (1989) J Devel Physiol 11: 37–43.

Sims ME, Beckwitt Turkell S, Halterman G, Paul RH (1985) Am J Obstet Gynecol 151: 721–723.

Vlessis AA and Mela-Riker L (1989) Ped Res 26: 220–226.

14

Human Fetal Haemodynamic Adaptation to Intrauterine Growth Retardation

G. P. MANDRUZZATO, P. BOGATTI, P. C. VEGLIO,
C. GIGLI, D. RUSTJA, R. CASACCIA AND L. FISHER

Divisione di Ostetrica e Ginecologia, Istituto per l'Infanzia, Trieste, Italy

Haemodynamic adaptation of the fetus to normal and abnormal conditions has been described in experimental animals and to a larger extent also in the human (Dawes, 1968). After the recent introduction of Doppler ultrasound methods, it has become much easier to investigate some characteristics of blood flow in human fetal and maternal vessels. By using real-time ultrasonic imaging equipment coupled with a Doppler probe it is possible to identify even small vessels, and to sample them to obtain clear measurements of blood flow velocity. Different indices, independent of the angle of insonation, can be calculated. The pulsatility index (PI) proposed by Gosling and Kind (1975) seems to be most informative. By measuring not only systolic and diastolic but also mean velocity the shape of the velocity waveform can be evaluated. It is therefore possible to obtain information related to the peripheral resistance of the vascular bed, which we have investigated.

In normal cases this resistance index (PI) is almost constant through pregnancy in the fetal thoracic descending aorta and internal carotid artery, and decreases in the umbilical artery as pregnancy progresses (Griffin et al., 1983; Wladimiroff et al., 1986; Bogatti et al., 1990). In abnormal conditions, such as intrauterine growth retardation (IUGR), in many cases PI values are increased in the aorta and umbilical artery and decreased in the internal carotid (Jouppila and Kirkinen, 1984; Giles et al., 1985). It has been postulated that an increased PI in the aorta is the effect of peripheral vasoconstriction, and the decrease in the cerebral vessels reflects the so-called 'brain sparing effect'. The augmented values of PI in the

Fetal Autonomy and Adaptation. Edited by G. S. Dawes, A. Zacutti, F. Borruto and A. Zacutti, Jr
© 1990 John Wiley & Sons Ltd

umbilical artery are considered to demonstrate an increase of the vascular resistance in the fetal placental circulation.

The aim of our study has been to investigate, by using pulsed Doppler velocimetry, how the fetus adapts its circulation with impaired growth in utero.

Materials and Methods

The study group consisted of 148 pregnancies in which serial ultrasonic measurements showed a reduction of fetal growth, as defined by biparietal diameter and/or abdominal circumference >2 SD below the mean values expected for gestational age. After recognition of IUGR, the maternal clinical condition was assessed and if necessary treated. At the same time the possibility of fetal chromosomal or structural abnormalities was investigated. Blood flow velocity waveforms were studied in the fetal descending aorta and umbilical artery, and usually also in the internal carotid, not less than weekly until delivery, according to the technique already described (Bogatti et al., 1989). The PI values were calculated and compared to our normal charts (Bogatti et al., 1990). The Doppler findings in the aorta and/or umbilical artery were considered abnormal when exceeding 2 SD from the mean, or with absent end-diastolic flow or with reverse flow in diastole. Observations on the internal carotid artery were considered abnormal when the PI was more than 2 SD below the mean.

The Doppler results were concealed from the clinician so as not to influence clinical decisions. The control of fetal conditions has been based on antepartum cardiotocography (CTG) using the non-stressed test (NST) and oxytocin challenge test (OCT). The diagnosis of fetal distress was based upon the observation of a non-reactive NST or positive OCT, *and* on the presence of late decelerations and/or fetal acidaemia in labour.

Results

Of the 148 fetuses showing growth retardation in utero, 108 were small for gestational age (SGA), having a birthweight below the 10th percentile of the Trieste population (Mandruzzato et al., 1973). Forty with a birthweight between the 10th and 25th percentile were defined as appropriate for gestational age (AGA). The incidence of fetal distress was 35.2% for the whole group, higher among SGA (37.9%) and lower in the AGA group (27.5%). The difference was not statistically significant (chi-squared = 1.40).

Abnormal Doppler findings were observed in 42.6% of the cases in the aorta, and in 20.9% in the umbilical artery. We never observed abnormal PI values in the umbilical artery with simultaneous normal values in the aorta. The sensitivity, specificity, and predictive values of abnormal Doppler

TABLE 1   Observations on 148 patients from Trieste: sensitivity, specificity, and values for predicting fetal distress* by a PI (pulsatility index) more than 2 SD above the mean in the fetal aorta or umbilical artery

	Fetal aorta	Umbilical artery
Sensitivity %	74.3	50.0
Specificity %	79.2	94.8
Predictive value positive test %	68.3	83.9
Predictive value negative test %	89.4	77.7

*As defined in Methods.

TABLE 2   Observations on the incidence of fetuses which were small (SGA) or appropriate (AGA) for gestational age, according to whether the pulsatility indices (PI) were abnormal (>2 SD from the mean) in the aorta and/or umbilical artery. Chi-squared = 1.19 (not significant)

Group abnormalities in:	1 Aorta and umbilical artery	2 Aorta only	3 None	Total
SGA	25 (23%)	23 (21.3%)	60 (55.6%)	108 (73%)
AGA	6 (15%)	9 (22.5%)	25 (62.5%)	40 (27%)
Total	31 (20.9%)	32 (21.6%)	85 (57.5%)	148

TABLE 3   Incidence of fetal distress (defined in methods) in 148 fetuses according to the pulsatility indices (PI) greater or less than 2 SD above the mean values in the fetal aorta and/or umbilical artery. Chi-squared = 59.3 ($p < 0.001$)

PI values	>2 SD AO+UA*		>2 SD AO:>2 SD UA		<2 SD AO+UA		Total	
Fetal distress present	26	84%	17	53%	9	10.5%	52	35%
Fetal distress absent	5	16%	15	47%	76	89.5%	96	65%
Total	31		32		85		148	

*AO = aorta; UA = umbilical artery.

findings for fetal distress are shown in Table 1 for the fetal aorta and umbilical artery.

The 148 cases were divided into three groups according to the Doppler findings. The first group comprised cases with abnormal PI values in *both* vessels; the second included those with abnormal PI values in the aorta only; and the third group consisted of those with normal values in both vessels. Table 2 shows the distribution of SGA and AGA fetuses between the three groups; the differences were not statistically significant. The frequency of fetal distress was significantly higher ($p < 0.001$) in the first group (with abnormal findings in both vessels; Table 3).

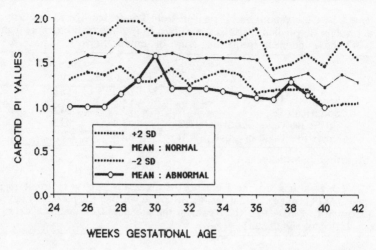

FIGURE 1   Changes with gestational age in the mean ($\pm$ SD) carotid PI values in normal fetuses, compared with those from fetuses in which both aortic and umbilical arterial PI values were abnormally elevated (open circles)

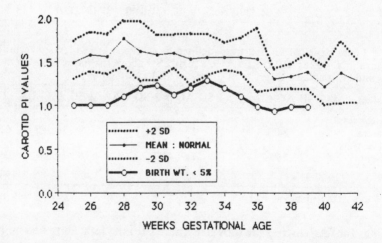

FIGURE 2   Changes with gestational age in the mean ($\pm$ SD) carotid PI values in normal fetuses, compared with those from fetuses in which both aortic and umbilical arterial PI values were abnormally elevated and there was severe intrauterine growth retardation (fetal wt. < 5th centile for age and sex on delivery, open circles)

Where available internal carotid PI values were usually 2 SD or more below the mean in the first group (Figure 1), and always abnormal when also associated with severe growth retardation (birthweight < 5th centile, Figure 2).

Discussion

Defective fetal growth can be the consequence of many factors related to maternal, fetal, or placental conditions. For a long time IUGR and SGA have been considered as being the same thing. Yet since the introduction of fetal ultrasonic biometry, it has become possible to observe the growth process longitudinally during intrauterine life; consideration of static birthweight as an indicator of IUGR has lost its importance. The frequency of fetal distress is similar in SGA and in AGA fetuses cases showing defective growth in utero. But even in this condition about 60% of fetuses can be delivered spontaneously without complications, since their reduced growth is not the consequence of a pathological condition (possibly) leading to hypoxia.

Measurement of haemodynamic patterns in fetuses with growth retardation not only differentiates the risk of developing fetal distress (Marsal and Persson, 1988; Mandruzzato et al., 1989), but also offers the opportunity of determining how the human fetus adapts its circulation to the possible stress of reduced placental exchange. Abnormal Doppler findings in the fetal descending thoracic aorta and umbilical artery may result from constriction of fetal vessels, with reduction of nutrient and gas exchange between mother and fetus. The reduction of resistance (lowered PI) in the carotid is believed to express the so-called 'brain sparing effect', an attempt to maintain oxygen supply to the cerebral tissues.

From the Doppler findings in the aorta and umbilical artery, we conclude that the haemodynamic response of IUGR fetuses is independent of birthweight, but related to the growth reduction process. Considering the relationship between haemodynamic patterns and abnormal CTG and/or fetal acidaemia (both believed to be related to the level of fetal oxygenation) the distribution is different in the three groups. In the third group, with no apparent haemodynamic involvement, the frequency of fetal hypoxia is low, about 10%. We suppose that this group of IUGR fetuses includes the vast majority of the so-called 'genetically small'. In the second group peripheral vasoconstriction is present but no abnormal values for the umbilical artery are found; the frequency of fetal distress is higher, about 50%. In these cases there may be some reduction of blood flow through the umbilical arteries, but not clearly identified using a cut-off point of 2 SD. In the first group where both vessels display abnormal values, the frequency of fetal distress is very high, more than 80%. In these cases redistribution of the fetal circulation is observed together with a large reduction of blood flow velocity in the umbilical artery, often leading to severe fetal hypoxia.

In the internal carotid artery abnormal PI values are constantly present only in extreme conditions: severe growth retardation (birthweight below the 5th centile) and systemic vasoconstriction together with considerable reduction of umbilical artery blood flow velocity.

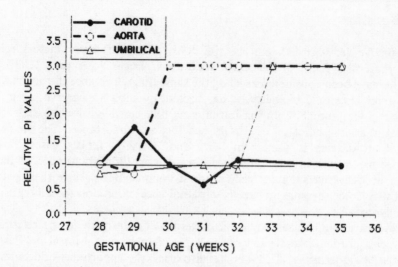

FIGURE 3   Changes in the pulsatility indices (PI values) with gestational age in a fetus with intrauterine growth retardation. For each observation the deviation from the outer limits of normality (mean + 2 SD for aorta and umbilical artery; mean − 2 SD for the carotid artery) is shown in order to illustrate the sequence of events

As to the mechanism of fetal adaptation to hypoxia, we might consider the chronological sequence in which abnormal values are observed in the different vascular beds. First, fetal systemic vasoconstriction (i.e. increased aortic PI values) always precedes the appearance of abnormal umbilical artery findings. The regulatory mechanisms of the fetal circulation may be more sensitive to variations in supply lines than our methods of investigation can detect.

We present one case of IUGR in which all the three vascular beds were evaluated longitudinally from the 28th gestational week until delivery, by caesarean section at 35 weeks gestational age (Figure 3). Abnormal values (> 2 SD above the mean) were present in the aorta from the 29th week onwards. In the internal carotid artery the values became abnormal by 30 weeks, and in the umbilical artery from 32 weeks onwards. This suggests that redistribution in the fetal circulation is modulated by very sensitive mechanisms, often as a response to stress rather than true fetal distress. The latter seems to appear only after a very large reduction of umbilical flow.

Conclusions

Pulsed Doppler evaluation of blood velocity waveforms offers useful information on the characteristics of the blood flow and peripheral resistance of the vascular beds concerned. Hence it is possible to study by a non-invasive technique longitudinally some aspects of fetal haemodynamic adaptation. We conclude as follows:

1. The fetus adapts its circulation following a sequence that seems related to the degree of the reduction of blood flow in the umbilical artery. Our methods are as yet inadequate to detect minor abnormalities.
2. From the clinical point of view this study of fetal haemodynamic adaptation may well offer information of value in defining more precisely the level of risk in fetuses with IUGR which may develop fetal hypoxia.

References

Bogatti P, Veglio PC, Rustja D, Mandruzzato GP (1989) Feto-placental haemodynamics in growth retardation: a pulsed Doppler study. Eur J Obstet Gynaecol & Reprod Biol 31: 213–219.

Bogatti P, Veglio PC, Rustja D, Mandruzzato GP, Alberico S (1990) Valori di normalita per l'indice di pulsatilita nei distretti arteriosi fetali e feto-placentari. Riv Ital di Ost Ginec e Med Perinatale (in press).

Dawes GS (1968) Fetal and Neonatal Physiology. Year Book Medical Publishers, Chicago.

Griffin D, Cohen Overbeek T, Campbell S (1983) Fetal and utero-placental blood flow. Clin Obstet Gynaecol 10: 566–600.

Giles W, Trudinger BJ, Baird PJ (1985) Fetal umbilical artery flow velocity waveforms and placental resistance: pathological correlation. Br Med J 92:31–38.

Gosling R and Kind D (1975) Arteries and veins. In: Ultrasound Angiology, p. 61. Churchill-Livingstone, Edinburgh.

Jouppila P and Kirkinen P (1984) Increased vascular resistance in the descending aorta of the fetus in hypoxia. Br J Obstet Gynaecol 91: 835–839.

Mandruzzato GP, Macagno F, Bellani R, Carli F, Carlomagno G, Sabbati MC (1973) Sul rapporto peso/eta gestazionale. Valutazione su 11701 nati. Ann Ost Gin Med Perinatale 94: 595.

Mandruzzato GP, Bogatti P, Veglio PC, Rustja D (1989) Umbilical artery and fetal aorta velocimetry in growth retarded fetuses. Rech Gynecol 1(5).

Marsal K and Persson P-H (1988) Ultrasonic measurement of fetal blood velocity wave form as a secondary diagnostic test in screening for intrauterine growth retardation. J Clin Ultrasound 16: 239–244.

Wladimiroff J, Tonge M, Stewart P (1986) Doppler ultrasound assessment of cerebral blood flow in the human fetus. Br Obstet Gynaecol 23: 471–475.

Discussion

Dawes asked whether the introduction of new technologies had changed the pattern of Gian Paulo's clinical behaviour. Mandruzzato replied that, to be honest, it had, even if there was still no clear evidence of the most appropriate clinical use of flow velocity waveform data, from umbilical or uterine arteries, for example. More controls were needed. Clinical adaptation must be gradual.

Clinical Application of Flow Velocity Waveform Data

Patrick asked whether, in sick growth-retarded fetuses, there was ever a *reversal* in the direction of change in the carotid diastolic:systolic ratio or pulsatility index (PI) as the fetus deteriorated. Mandruzzato replied that in two cases the carotid PI had fallen very low, to pathological limits, and then rose terminally as the fetus deteriorated further, suggesting perhaps a fall in arterial pressure, or at least the inability of the fetus to sustain the brain sparing effect.

Patrick also raised the issue of using Doppler flow studies on the fetus (aorta or umbilical arteries) or mother (uterine arteries) as a possible screening test, as advocated by some in the USA and Australia (e.g. Trudinger et al., 1987). Mandruzzato replied that the method was advocated by Stuart Campbell, to suggest increased resistance in the arcuate or uterine arteries at 20–24 weeks gestation in association with increased risk of pregnancy complications such as hypertension and abruption. As yet there was no clear evidence as to whether this was useful as a screening test; the majority view was against it. The method was useful in the investigation of high-risk pregnancies. Ianniruberto ('Fetus as Patient' Conference, Bari, September 1988) had examined 2000 pregnant women, using a simple inexpensive continuous wave Doppler examination of the umbilical artery, suitable for use by a midwife, in search for evidence of fetal distress. But in Mandruzzato's opinion this should be carried out after good ultrasound screening of fetal growth. Pardi agreed; it was uncertain as yet how much weight should be attached to this data in determining the appropriate time for delivery.

Both he and Marsal (Marsal, 1988) divided growth-retarded babies into two groups: one with a high probability of developing fetal distress as determined by changes in heart rate, treated intensively in hospital; the other followed each week in the clinic by FHR monitoring and ultrasound examination, none of which had been lost by intrauterine death. In 12 of 148 infants so studied the pulsatility index had risen greatly, and in some records end-diastolic flow was absent. More evidence was needed to understand the significance of this phenomenon.

Pardi asked about the results as to neurological outcome. Mandruzzato explained that 17 of the 128 infants were lost to follow-up. He was surprised that there was no major neurological abnormality (using the criteria of Touwen et al., 1980) in the remainder after 6–36 months, in spite of the high incidence of abnormal Doppler flow measurements (PI values abnormal in both aorta and umbilical artery and absent end-diastolic flow: 12 patients).

Patrick pointed out that the published data showed that in very high-risk pregnancies (3%) the absolute figures for perinatal mortality and morbidity were small. Most cases of gross neurological abnormality, including cerebral palsy, occurred in the 85% of patients with low-risk pregnancies; it was these which attracted law suits. Barker pointed out that the same was true of Down's syndrome: the incidence was higher in older women, but most of the infants with Down's syndrome have young mothers. Mandruzzato agreed that this was true of almost anything in obstetrics; 80% of fetal malformations and 60% of growth retardation came from low-risk groups. It seemed that discrimination was not very decisive.

Evaluation of Fetal Flow Velocity Data

Pardi asked whether many, or any, symmetrically growth-retarded fetuses can have an abnormal pulsatility index (PI) in the umbilical arteries. Mandruzzato thought this was possible, because he had seen three infants (one with trisomy 21 and two with trisomy 18) with abnormal PI values and severe symmetrical growth retardation, though it was nowadays unusual to find such cases late in gestation. Pardi considered that growth retardation might occur with karyotype abnormalities only at the level of the placental trophoblast, perhaps leading to inappropriate invasion of the endometrium.

Redman returned to a critique of flow velocity waveform evaluation, asking whether abnormalities of waveforms in the aorta precede the appearance of those in the umbilical arteries, and hence whether the aorta need be studied at all. Mandruzzato replied that when both umbilical and aortic waveforms were abnormal the chance of subsequent fetal distress was 85%; with an aortic abnormality only the chance was 53%; with an umbilical arterial abnormality only the chance was 10%. Dawes asked whether both umbilical arteries were studied, and Redman said it was possible to get dissimilar readings; in one published case (Trudinger and Cook, 1988) flow was abnormal in one artery, with poor diastolic flow in the other, which supplied an infarcted area of placenta. [Since then seven more cases have been recorded of discordant umbilical artery flow velocity waveforms; Harper and Murnaghan, 1989: Ed] Pardi said that only one umbilical artery was sampled in his laboratory; he assumed physiological anastomosis between the two vessels but thought it would be interesting to seek differences by colour Doppler velocimetry.

In reply to a question from Zacutti, Mandruzzato said that comparison of results from computerized CTG analysis and other biophysical measurements (e.g. flow velocity waveforms) was still in progress. There was a good relation between the reduction in long-term FHR variation (mean range of fetal pulse interval variation) and abnormal (Doppler) flow velocity waveform findings. In his view the computerized CTG system was cheaper and easier to use. In a couple of years time, with increased knowledge, it might be possible to stop using the more expensive Doppler equipment; colour Doppler equipment was expensive but it had the advantage of identifying vessels quickly, even when small, and giving more precise information on flow velocity. But its use cannot be justified outside research centres as yet.

Growth Retardation: Biological Variation and Mathematical Models

Finally, there was a brief discussion on the logical distinction between normal variatior and pathological change. Barker found the definition of intrauterine growth retardation, as a percentile, difficult to accept. He quoted the distribution of values of serum cholesterol in Great Britain, where the whole distribution of values was elevated as compared with some other countries. Hence average values in Britain are usual but not normal. Dawes agreed. It had to be established, in each instance, whether the fetuses 2 SD or more from the mean were truly abnormal, judged by a definite medical or biological criterion. The statistical model was crude and unreliable. This issue was important; the common assumption that a particular centile was a valid criterion needed testing. Redman also agreed; he argued that the ideal growth curve was not necessarily applicable to a particular fetus, each of which had its own target.

References

Harper MA and Murnaghan GA (1989) Br J Obstet Gynaecol 96: 1449–1452.
Marsal K (1988) J Clin Ultrasound 16: 239.
Touwen BCL, Huisjes HJ, Jurgens-van der Zee AD et al. (1980) Early Human Dev 4: 207.
Trudinger BJ, Cook CM, Giles WB et al. (1987) Lancet i: 188–190.
Trudinger BJ and Cook CM (1988) Obstet Gynecol 71: 1019–1021.

Conclusion

Dawes concluded by thanking Professor Alberto Zacutti, on behalf of the participants, for suggesting the meeting and making it possible. He asked him to convey their gratitude to all his colleagues, the sponsors, and the secretariat. It had been a great privilege to come to such a beautiful place and to be given the leisure for a free-ranging and speculative discussion on fetal autonomy and adaptation. The mixture of basic and clinical science had been especially profitable, and had raised important issues, both practical and academic, for future research.

Fetal Autonomy and Adaptation. Edited by G. S. Dawes, A. Zacutti, F. Borruto and A. Zacutti, Jr
© 1990 John Wiley & Sons Ltd

Index